Principles of Operative Dentistry

A.J.E. Qualtrough
J.D. Satterthwaite
L.A. Morrow
P.A. Brunton

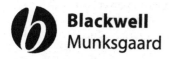
Blackwell
Munksgaard

© 2005 by A.J.E. Qualtrough, J.D. Satterthwaite, L.A. Morrow and P.A. Brunton

Blackwell Munksgaard, a Blackwell Publishing company
Editorial Offices:
Blackwell Publishing Ltd, 9600 Garsington Road, Oxford OX4 2DQ, UK
  Tel: +44 (0)1865 776868
Blackwell Publishing Professional, 2121 State Avenue, Ames, Iowa 50014-8300, USA
  Tel: +1 515 292 0140
Blackwell Publishing Asia Pty Ltd, 550 Swanston Street, Carlton, Victoria 3053, Australia
  Tel: +61 (0)3 8359 1011

First published 2005 by Blackwell Munksgaard

Library of Congress Cataloging-in-Publication Data
Principles of operative dentistry / A.J.E. Qualtrough . . . [et al.].
    p. ; cm.
Includes bibliographical references and index.
ISBN-13: 978-1-4051-1821-7 (pbk. : alk. paper)
ISBN-10: 1-4051-1821-0 (pbk. : alk. paper)
1. Dentistry, Operative. 2. Endodontics. 3. Evidence-based dentistry.
I. Qualtrough, A. J. E.
[DNLM: 1. Dentistry, Operative–methods. 2. Endodontics–methods.
3. Evidence-Based Medicine.   WU 300 P9575 2005]
RK501.P854 2005
617.6′05–dc22

2004026345

ISBN-13: 978-1-4051-1821-7
ISBN-10: 1-4051-1821-0

A catalogue record for this title is available from the British Library

Set in 10/13 pt Palatino
by Graphicraft Limited, Hong Kong

For further information on Blackwell Munksgaard, visit our website:
www.dentistry.blackwellmunksgaard.com

Contents

Foreword   v
Preface   vii
Contributors   ix
Acknowledgements   x

1 **Basic principles**   1
   Ergonomics in dentistry   1
   Examination of the dentition – occlusion   8
   Examination of the dentition – charting   11
   Dental caries   14
   Moisture control   19

2 **Principles of direct intervention**   27
   Preservative management   27
   Principles of operative intervention   27
   Alternative preparation methods   33
   Pulp protection   36
   Supplementary retention for direct restorations   43

3 **Principles of endodontics**   51
   Introduction   51
   Diagnosis and assessment   52
   Endodontic imaging   54
   Access cavities   56
   Endodontic instruments   62
   Cleaning and shaping   68
   Inter-appointment medicaments   73
   Obturation (root filling)   75

4 **Endodontics – further considerations**   81
   Trauma   81
   Perio-endo connections   86
   Elective endodontics   90
   Restoration of the root-filled tooth   93

5 **Principles of indirect restoration**   107
   Introduction and indications   107
   Core restorations   111
   Principles of preparation for indirect restorations   115
   Summary   127

6 **Indirect restorations – further considerations**   129
   Material type   129
   Intra/extra-coronal restoration   133
   Partial coverage restorations   133
   Temporisation   134
   Impression taking   139
   Methods of construction   143
   Limited resistance and retention   145
   Creation of interocclusal space   147
   Limitations of indirect restorations   150

7 **Maintenance of the restored dentition**   153
   Maintenance   153
   Failure   154
   Replacement and repair of restorations   156

8 **Evidence based practice**   161
   Introduction – what is evidence based practice?   161
   Identifying and defining relevant questions   162
   Identifying evidence   163
   Appraisal of research literature   167
   Implementation of research evidence and evaluation
      of its application   170
   Conclusion   171

   Index   173

Foreword

Operative dentistry forms the central part of dentistry as practised in primary care. It occupies the majority of a dentist's working life and is a key component of restorative dentistry. It is unfortunate that the academic discipline of operative dentistry has become less clearly identifiable within many dental schools. The Operative Dentistry or Conservative Dentistry Department is now often part of a larger department of Restorative Dentistry and can less easily be seen as a discipline in its own right. Indeed, operative dentistry is not recognised as a specialty either in the United Kingdom or the United States which, given its central position in the delivery of oral healthcare to patients, is unfortunate.

The subject of operative dentistry continues to evolve rapidly as the improved understanding of the aetiology and prevention of the common dental diseases is linked with advances in restorative techniques and materials. The effective practice of operative dentistry requires not only excellent manual skills but an understanding of both the disease processes affecting teeth and the properties of the materials available for their restoration.

In view of the seemingly diminished status of operative dentistry, it is all the more pleasing that four well-known, younger academic and hospital-based colleagues have collaborated to create this new book, *Principles of Operative Dentistry*. It is directed primarily towards the dental undergraduate but will benefit the primary care dentist as well as those engaged in more formal postgraduate study. Many operative textbooks place an emphasis on technique but sometimes do not describe adequately the thinking that underpins both the operative procedures and the overall management of the patient. The authors are to be commended for having taken the logical approach of examining the reasons for the procedures and techniques available in operative dentistry. There is wide coverage of the subject, including the restoration of cavities in teeth, management of the dental pulp, the various types of indirect restorations and the management of failed restorations.

The clear presentation and easy style of the book encourages the reader, whilst the arguments for and against particular techniques are supported by reference to the dental literature. The latter is of increasing importance as the demand for evidence-based dentistry gains momentum. The inclusion of a chapter explaining evidence-based practice and how information can be found is particularly welcome. This book provides a wealth of information which is a distillation of the knowledge and experience of the authors. It is also a book for the reader to enjoy and it is to be hoped that it will stimulate a life-long interest in the principles and practice of operative dentistry.

Richard Ibbetson
Director, Edinburgh Postgraduate Dental Institute
and Professor of Primary Dental Care, University of Edinburgh

Preface

Operative dentistry is a significant part of clinical dentistry, with practitioners in the UK spending more than 60% of their time placing and replacing direct restorations. In tandem with this many root canal treatments are carried out and increasingly more indirect restorations are placed. All practitioners whatever their discipline will remember developing their manual skills while engaged in these procedures during their student days.

This book is about the theoretical concepts that underpin clinical practice in the areas of operative dentistry and endodontology and it is primarily directed at clinical dental students and professionals complementary to dentistry. The aim of the text is to provide students with the knowledge required while they are developing the necessary clinical skills and attitudes in their undergraduate training in operative dentistry and endodontology. It is specifically designed to be read in conjunction with pre-clinical and clinical training.

Each chapter addresses various aspects of the subject and there is directed additional reading in the form of selected relevant references. Specific tips will be highlighted throughout the text and there is information about the application of dental materials, although readers are referred to specific texts on dental materials for further information.

After reading this book the reader should be able to:

- Sit properly while operating and be able to organise their operating environment effectively
- Chart teeth
- Understand the basics of cariology, specifically diagnose caries more effectively especially in its early stages
- Prepare teeth to include supplementary retention if indicated clinically
- Understand modern pulp protection regimes
- Select and place the correct restorative material
- Understand when endodontic treatment is indicated
- Access the pulp chamber and root canal systems of teeth

- Effectively clean, shape and obturate the root canal system
- Restore endodontically treated teeth
- Determine when indirect restorations are indicated
- Prepare teeth appropriately for indirect restorations
- Manage soft tissues and use impression materials
- Place a variety of temporary restorations
- Select restorations suitable for repair and refurbishment procedures

Increasingly the evidence base for dentistry is being challenged and it is often said that only 15% of the whole of dentistry is evidence based. The book therefore concludes with a chapter on evidence based dentistry, as the practitioners of the future must have a working knowledge of the principles of evidence based care.

Contributors

Julian D. Satterthwaite BDS MSc MFDS FDSRCS(Eng)
Lecturer in Restorative Dentistry, School of Dentistry, University of Manchester, UK

Leean A. Morrow BDS(Hons) MPhil FDS FDS(Rest Dent) RCS(Eng)
Consultant in Restorative Dentistry, The Leeds Teaching Hospitals NHS Trust, Leeds, UK

Alison J.E. Qualtrough BChD MSc PhD FDS MRDRCS(Edin)
Senior Lecturer/Honorary Consultant in Restorative Dentistry, School of Dentistry, University of Manchester, UK

Paul A. Brunton BChD MSc PhD FDS FDS(Rest Dent) RCS(Eng)
Professor/Honorary Consultant in Restorative Dentistry, Leeds Dental Institute, University of Leeds, UK

Evidence based care
Helen Worthington MSc PhD
Professor of Evidence Based Care/Coordinating Editor of Cochrane Oral Health Group, School of Dentistry, University of Manchester, UK

Anne-Marie Glenny MMedSci
Lecturer in Evidence Based Oral Health Care, School of Dentistry, University of Manchester, UK

Ergonomics
W. Alan Hopwood BDS MDS
Clinical Teacher in Restorative Dentistry, School of Dentistry, University of Manchester, UK

Radiology
Keith Horner BChD MSc PhD FDSRCPS(Glasg) FRCR DDR
Professor of Oral and Maxillofacial Imaging/Honorary Consultant in Dental and Maxillofacial Radiology, School of Dentistry, University of Manchester, UK

Illustrations
Raymond Evans MAA RMIP, Medical Illustrator

Acknowledgements

We would like to express our gratitude to all those individuals who have been formative to the ethos of teaching at the School of Dentistry, University of Manchester. This philosophy was the stimulus for the production of this text. Although many individuals have been involved, we are particularly grateful to Professor Nairn Wilson and Drs John Lilley and Shaun Whitehead.

In addition, we would like to express our thanks to Mr Clive Atack, Chief Photographer, Unit of Medical Illustration, School of Dentistry, University of Manchester, for Figs 1.2 to 1.5.

Basic principles

ERGONOMICS IN DENTISTRY

Ergonomics is defined as 'the study of man in relation to his working environment: the adaptation of machines and general conditions to fit the individual so that he may work at maximum efficiency'.

The application of these principles concerns every aspect of design within the building and streamlining of procedure. Within the surgery, the contemporary dental unit is a masterpiece of design incorporating as many ergonomic features as possible to enable the operator, dental nurse and patient to experience the minimum of stress and fatigue. It is evident, furthermore, that this environment must facilitate a high standard of dental treatment as clinical techniques become ever more complex and exacting.

This transformation began with the general adoption of a comfortable, supported and seated position for the operator and the consequent supine positioning of the patient. However, the necessary changes in posture and working procedures were largely overlooked and, despite the convincing work and publication of Paul[1], it would seem that many dentists persist in working in inefficient, distorted postures that must frequently lead to excessive fatigue if not skeletal damage.

The operator's chair

This should be fully adjustable and mobile, provide a broad, preferably anatomically contoured seat and give support in the lumbar region. It should be adjusted in height to suit each individual operator in order to distribute the weight equally between the thighs and feet. The dental nurse chair differs only, but importantly, in that it must adjust to at least a 10 cm increase in height and provide a corresponding 'bar stool' type rim rest for the feet.

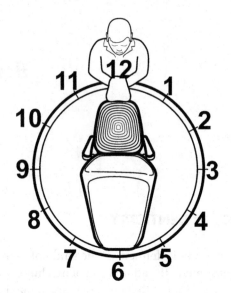

Fig. 1.1 Position of operator relative to chair.

Operator and nurse positions

The dentist will normally work within a range from the 12 o'clock to the 9 o'clock position relative to the patient's head. However, most operative procedures are completed from, at, or near, the 12 o'clock position. The dental nurse will normally remain in a fixed position at 4 o'clock (Fig. 1.1) but at a considerably higher position in order to look down or forward to the mouth. This height not only facilitates the different tasks, but enables the nurse to visualise the back of the mouth and remove any accumulation of debris or water.

Operator's vision

There can be no doubt that any tooth is best visualised by direct vision (Fig. 1.2). However, the nature of operative dentistry demands that, whenever possible, the line of vision is perpendicular to the tooth surface. Clearly, those surfaces inaccessible by direct vision must be visualised indirectly through a mirror (Fig. 1.3). Nevertheless, it remains important, however difficult, to position the mirror and attempt a near perpendicular view. Magnification of the working area provides a major advantage in both the reduction of eye strain and the promotion of high standards.

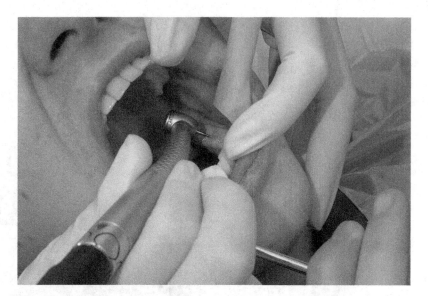

Fig. 1.2 Direct vision.

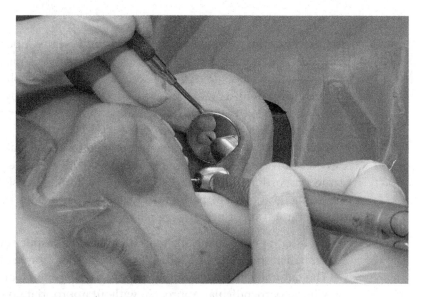

Fig. 1.3 Visualisation in mirror.

Patient position

Adoption of the supine patient position by most dental practitioners has focused attention on the optimal position of the patient's head in relation to the seated operator. Paul[1] compares this relationship in

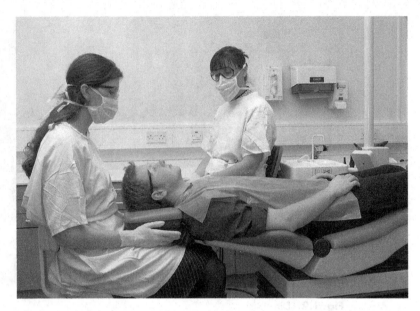

Fig. 1.4 The home position.

dentistry to any other precision activity by a seated operator and describes the 'home position' in which the objective is raised to the mid-sternal position and the head tilted forward to observe the fingers. Most dentists will gradually adopt this position by trial and error and indeed many will programme the dental chair to return and permit this situation for every patient (Fig. 1.4).

Observation of a large number of operators over many years reveals, however, that for some procedures, with a supine patient, a large proportion will adopt distinctly uncomfortable, distorted and fatiguing positions. Furthermore, it would appear that the reasons for this distortion are principally related to:

- An attempt to adopt a direct visual approach, despite severe postural distortion, when an indirect approach is more appropriate.
- The natural, almost in-built attempt to visualise the tooth surface via the perpendicular approach, without appropriate positioning and rotation of the patient's head.

The former situation should be corrected by training, practice and a disciplined procedure but the latter can only be corrected by a different patient posture provided by a modified chair position. Specifically, the difficulty lies in viewing the lower posterior teeth in the fully supine patient. In this situation, it can undoubtedly be an

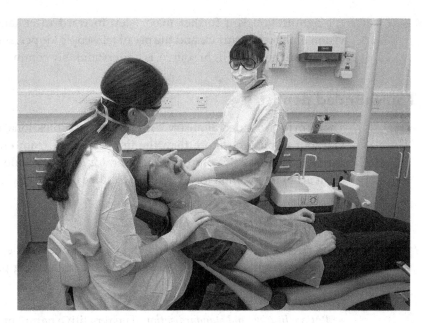

Fig. 1.5 The home position for lower teeth.

advantage to position the chair base considerably lower but tilted forward to approximately 40° from the waist to return the patient's head to the 'home' position (Fig. 1.5). The correctly seated operator will have a visual approach near perpendicular to the posterior surfaces.

Illumination

There can be no better illustration of the recent transformation in working procedures than in the area of illumination. Indeed, it is a tribute to the dentists of the past that they accomplished such complex tasks with little other than an anglepoise lamp.

The enormous advantage of halogen unit lamps is self-evident. No doubt the future will prove even brighter with light emitting diodes (LEDs). In addition, the increasing use of fibre-optic handpieces ensures constantly focused illumination of the working area and eliminates the need to use the mirror as an additional aid to reflect unit-sourced light. Despite these advances, when using light-sensitive materials such as resin composites, it remains necessary to work with low light levels as high intensity light will lead to premature polymerisation of the material, thus preventing manipulation.

Magnification is a further major step forward in enhancing the vision of the work surface and the use of telescopic loupes, sometimes fitted with their own light source, is understandably commonplace.

Four-handed dentistry

The term four-handed dentistry is now rooted in professional terminology but implies no more than the importance of team effort. The dental team normally comprises the operator and nurse (four hands), but it is not uncommon for an additional nurse to make six.

Principles of four-handed dentistry

There are many ways in which the dental team can work efficiently, along ergonomic principles. Nevertheless, the underlying principles are:

- *Rationalisation and standardisation.* The repetitive nature of so much in dentistry offers the ideal opportunity to ration the immediate supply of instruments to those most commonly used and, also, to standardise technique so that, with practice, considerably greater efficiency will be achieved.

- *Delegation.* Delegation is the transfer of any task to a person who is both qualified and capable. This remains an area in which many dentists fail to take full advantage of the skills of the dental nurse.

- *Anticipation.* The experienced dental nurse will quickly learn the individual methods of the operator and begin to anticipate almost every situation. As a member of a regular dental team, rather than one based on rotational duty, the advantages can be significant.

- *Safety.* The focus and control achieved in all the various approaches to four-handed dentistry is undoubtedly matched by improved safety for both patient and operator. However, while there has been understandable concern that a supine patient may be at greater risk of ingestion or inhalation of foreign matter, it has been shown that, in this position, the tongue rests against the soft palate to provide a seal[2]. Nevertheless, some posterior pooling of fluid will inevitably occur and the responsibility of both nurse and operator in the control and removal of this accumulation cannot be overstated.

  In procedures carrying higher risk, such as endodontics, the total protection of the airway utilising rubber dam is self-evident.

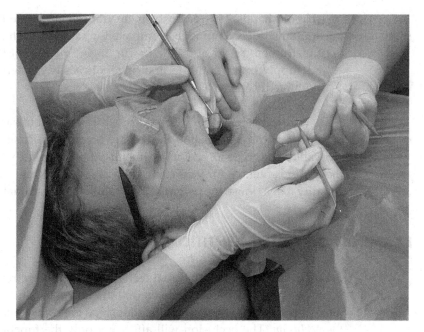

Fig. 1.6 Exchange of instruments in the transfer zone.

However, it is essential that no dental procedure should take place without appropriate airway protection, irrespective of patient position.

All patients, and indeed members of the dental team, should be provided with protective eyewear and for the supine patient, no transfer of materials or instruments should occur over the face.

- *Methods.* The concept of four-handed, ergonomic dentistry is open to varied individual approach and has been described in detail by Paul[1]. However, the underlying principle demands that all delivery, discard and transfer takes place in the area of safety and convenience around and below the chin – the so-called 'transfer zone' (Fig. 1.6). This practice demands maximal delegation to the dental nurse and requires concerted effort and understanding. However, the advantage to the operator, and hence the patient, of an undistracted focus on the tooth is considerable.

A comparison is with that of the general surgeon awaiting the appropriate instrument, correctly positioned for immediate grasp and use. The dentist's hands should therefore remain whenever possible in the transfer zone, instruments and materials should be asked for, not looked for, and be received to enable correct grasp with no risk of injury.

If both hands are free, instrument transfer is simple but more commonly the task must be completed in one hand. This method of instrument retrieval by the fourth finger, rotation of the wrist, and supply from thumb to first fingers is easily mastered and is undoubtedly efficient.

Therefore, it is clear that when due attention is paid to basic procedural aspects and organisation, the clinical scenario is efficient, effective, enjoyable and professional. On the other hand, without such discipline, there is the potential for inefficiency, lower standards and a lost opportunity to maximise the potential for a fulfilled professional career.

EXAMINATION OF THE DENTITION – OCCLUSION

Before examining any individual teeth that may require restoration, it is important to look at all the teeth, how they meet and how they move against each other. These relationships are collectively termed the *occlusion*. The occlusion will affect not only the functional load to which a tooth or restoration is subjected, but can also influence the shape and form of a restoration. For example, if a molar tooth is separated by a considerable amount from its antagonist tooth during movement of the mandible, than there is plenty of height for cusps to be carved into a restoration. Conversely, if restoring a tooth that rubs against its antagonist during movement of the mandible, then cusps are likely to be more shallow, and care must be taken that excess load is not placed onto the restoration during function.

Preoperative examination of the occlusion is essential. Note must be taken of existing relationships, both static and dynamic/excursive. The use of thin articulating paper to mark the teeth and identify contacts is required. Differing colours may be used for static and dynamic contacts. Study models, mounted with a face bow record on an articulator, may also prove to be useful, especially if multiple units or units involving guiding surfaces are to be restored. An explanation of occlusal terminology and relationships follows.

Intercuspal position (ICP)

The intercuspal position is the static position of maximum interdigitation of the cusps of the teeth, where the mandible is in its most closed position: it is also an habitual position. This position may be easily reproducible and identified on study models as 'best fit' (e.g. in a fully dentate patient) or may be difficult to identify and perhaps variable (e.g. in a patient with tooth wear). It is a *changeable and unstable position* as it will change as the teeth change throughout the lifetime of the patient. It is also called *maximum interdigitation position (MIP)* and *centric occlusion (CO)*.

Retruded axis position (RAP)

The retruded axis position is not a fixed point, but an 'arc' defined by the movement of the mandible when retruded, at which only hinge movements are possible. It is also called *terminal hinge axis* or *centric relation (CR)*. RAP is also defined anatomically as the position where the condyles are most superiorly placed within the glenoid fossae, with the articular discs in a close-packed position. It is a relaxed relationship and is the only true reproducible position.

Retruded contact position (RCP)

The retruded contact position is the point of first contact (between a maxillary and mandibular tooth) when closing on the retruded arc of closure (see RAP above). The movement from the RCP to ICP is termed a *slide*, and note should be taken of the magnitude of this slide as well as direction (i.e. vertical, horizontal – anterior to posterior and lateral components).

Excursion/excursive movements

Excursion relates to the dynamic movements of the mandible, as in:

- *Lateral excursion* – to the side (left or right)
- *Protrusion* – forward/anterior movement of the mandible
- *Retrusion* – backward/posterior movement of the mandible

Working side

The working side is the side to which the mandible moves when making a lateral excursive movement.

Non-working side

The non-working side is the opposite side from that to which the mandible moves when making a lateral excursive movement. Sometimes called the *balancing* or *orbiting* side.

Anterior/posterior determinants and guidance

Determinants of mandibular movements are the influences determining the envelope of possible movements of the mandible. These influences may be:

- *Posterior determinants* (i.e. the temporomandibular joints and anatomical structures associated with them, also termed *condylar guidance/posterior guidance*).
- *Anterior determinants* (i.e. the teeth).

The tooth surfaces that are in contact during an excursive movement are said to 'guide' movement of the mandible. The type of guidance may be divided as below, the divisions broadly describing the teeth that provide the guiding surface:

- *Anterior guidance* – the tooth surfaces that are in contact during a protrusive excursion. This is normally the incisor teeth, and hence is then termed *incisal guidance*: in some cases (for example an occlusion with an anterior open bite) it may actually be the posterior occlusal tooth surfaces that provide the anterior guidance.
- *Canine guidance* – when a lateral excursion is made, the canines on the working side are the only teeth to make contact.
- *Group function* – when a lateral excursion is made, multiple pairs of teeth on the working side make contact.

Tooth contacts during dynamic excursive movements that do not provide a smooth guidance, or separate guiding surfaces, may be termed an *interference*.

Non-working contact

A non-working contact is a contact between a pair of tooth surfaces on the non-working side during an excursive movement that does *not* otherwise interfere with the smooth movement of the mandible nor cause the guiding surfaces on the working side to be separated.

Non-working interference (NWI)

A non-working interference is a contact between a pair of tooth surfaces on the non-working side, during an excursive movement, that *interferes* with the smooth movement of the mandible and/or causes the guiding surfaces on the working side to be separated. It is important to identify such contacts as they are thought to cause high lateral loads on teeth and a subsequent predisposition to mechanical failure of a restoration.

Any new restoration must be in harmony with the existing occlusion if this is satisfactory. Where occlusal contacts are present that may cause treatment difficulties or a predisposition to failure, then steps should be taken to address this. For example, a cavity margin might be extended to avoid a contact at the potentially weak tooth-restoration interface or a non-working side interference reduced or eliminated (Chapter 2). Similarly, where indirect restorations are planned, these may be used to create a new occlusal relationship in situations when the existing pattern is not satisfactory.

EXAMINATION OF THE DENTITION – CHARTING

A dental charting is a stylised record of the patient's current dental status. It is good clinical practice to record the dental status at initial presentation and subsequent follow-up appointments. A full dental charting should be recorded in all patients' notes, thus forming part of the medico-legal record. It is not necessary to map the patient's restorations in detail on the charting, it is sufficient to record the type of restoration and/or cavity, not its exact dimensional extent. The object of a dental chart is to record:

- All teeth present.
- Teeth that are absent or unerupted.
- Presence and condition of existing restorations (including partial dentures and bridgework).
- Presence and extent of dental caries and other dental abnormalities, (e.g. non-carious tooth tissue loss, fractures, developmental defects and discoloration).

Tooth notation

Several different systems are available for tooth reference; there are however three systems that most practitioners should be aware of in order to be familiar with the increasing internationalisation of dental journals, conferences and other forms of communication. Most systems divide the mouth into four quadrants, which are indicated as if one is viewing the patient from the front:

upper right	upper left
lower right	lower left

Palmer system

The permanent teeth are numbered from 1 to 8, from central incisor to third molar. Each tooth also has be identified by the quadrant, thus the upper right first permanent molar is designated 6|, while the upper left first permanent molar is designated |6:

Patient's right   87654321 | 12345678   Patient's left

                         87654321 | 12345678

The primary (deciduous) teeth are represented by the letters A to E, from central incisor to second deciduous molar and also have to have a quadrant designation e.g. the upper right deciduous central incisor is A|.

Patient's right   EDCBA | ABCDE   Patient's left

                         EDCBA | ABCDE

It is advisable to use capital letters when referring to the deciduous dentition using the Palmer notation. If lower case letters are used, b can look like 6, and vice versa. This is especially important when patients are being referred for dental extractions.

Federation Dentaire Internationale (FDI) system

This system is commonly used in Europe. Each tooth is given a two-digit number; the first digit identifies the quadrant in which the tooth is situated and the second digit identifies the tooth in that quadrant.

In the permanent dentition, the quadrants are numbered from 1 to 4 starting with the upper right, which is quadrant 1, and continuing round in a clockwise direction to the lower right, which is quadrant 4. The teeth are numbered from 1 to 8 in each quadrant starting with 1 being the central incisor and continuing to 8 being the 3rd permanent molar. The permanent dentition is:

      Quadrant 1   Quadrant 2

18 17 16 15 14 13 12 11 | 21 22 23 24 25 26 27 28

48 47 46 45 44 43 42 41 | 31 32 33 34 35 36 37 38

      Quadrant 4   Quadrant 3

In the deciduous dentition, the quadrants are numbered from 5 to 8 starting with the upper right, which is quadrant 5, and continuing round in a clockwise direction to the lower right, which is quadrant 8. The teeth are numbered from 1 to 5 in each quadrant starting with 1 being the central incisor and continuing to 5 being the second deciduous molar. The deciduous dentition is:

Quadrant 5	Quadrant 6
55 54 53 52 51	61 62 63 64 65
85 84 83 82 81	71 72 73 74 75
Quadrant 8	Quadrant 7

Universal system

This system is commonly used in America. The teeth are given individual numbers from 1 to 32, starting with the upper right third molar and moving clockwise round the arch to the lower right third molar.

1 2 3 4 5 6 7 8	9 10 11 12 13 14 15 16
32 31 30 29 28 27 26 25	24 23 22 21 20 19 18 17

Surfaces of teeth

When describing a cavity or restoration, the location can be described by the surfaces of the tooth that are involved. These are as follows:

- Mesial: nearest to the midline of dental arch
- Distal: further from the midline of dental arch
- Labial: next to lips (anterior teeth)
- Buccal: next to cheeks (posterior teeth)
- Lingual: next to tongue (lower teeth)
- Palatal: next to palate (upper teeth)
- Incisal: cutting edge of anterior teeth
- Occlusal: chewing surface of posterior teeth

These surfaces can be represented diagrammatically as a box with five areas, each of which represents a surface (Fig. 1.7). A series of such boxes is used to represent all of the teeth (Fig. 1.8).

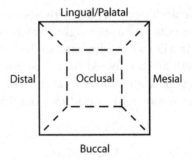

Fig. 1.7 Representation of tooth surface.

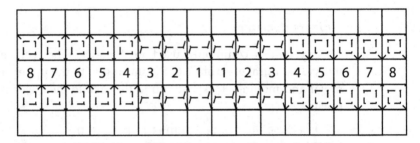

Fig. 1.8 Typical charting matrix.

DENTAL CARIES

Dental caries is a disease process resulting in the demineralisation of dental hard tissues by microbial activity. It is a readily preventable disease and can be arrested or reversed in its early stages. The pattern of dental caries has changed in recent years; new lesions are more likely to develop in pits and fissures, with smooth surface lesions becoming less common[3].

Aetiology

Dental caries has a multifactorial aetiology; however four principle factors are necessary for the production of a carious lesion:

- Bacteria in dental plaque
- Substrate such as a fermentable carbohydrate (dietary sugars)
- A susceptible tooth surface
- Time

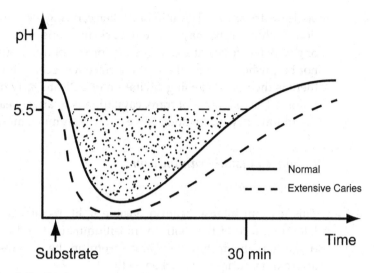

Fig. 1.9 Stephan curve.

Elimination of one or more of these factors is required for the prevention of dental caries. There is no single test that can take into consideration all the above factors and accurately predict an individual's susceptibility to caries. The diet type and frequency of intake is thought to play a significant role in the carious process. Bacteria in the dental plaque are capable of fermenting suitable carbohydrate substrates to produce acid, causing the pH to fall within minutes, resulting in demineralisation of the tooth tissue[4]. The plaque remains acidic for some time, taking 30–60 min to return to its normal pH in the region of 7. These changes in pH can be represented graphically over a period of time following a glucose rinse, which is frequently referred to as a Stephan curve (Fig. 1.9). The shaded area represents the risk of carious attack to the tooth surface: this area is larger in a patient with extensive caries.

Caries diagnosis and assessment

As with all diagnostic tests, there is the potential for operator error, therefore careful interpretation is required.

Visual examination

Visual inspection of the tooth is the first and most widely used method; however it may be surprisingly inaccurate. The tooth must be clean, dry and well illuminated when carrying out a visual examination. A blunt probe may be useful to clean debris off the tooth surface or gently feel for cavities; however, a probe, blunt or otherwise, must not be pushed against the tooth surface (especially into fissures) as there is the risk of causing cavitation of delicate early demineralised lesions. The diagnosis of frank cavitation is relatively easy, but slight discoloration, which is suggestive of caries, is much more difficult.

Enhanced visual examination

Transillumination

This uses an intense beam of visible light, usually directed on the lateral surface of the tooth to transilluminate it and aid with caries diagnosis. This technique is most useful in the diagnosis of anterior approximal caries and cracked teeth.

Fibre-optic transillumination

This technique uses a fibre-optic light source placed palatal to anterior teeth to aid diagnosis of anterior approximal caries. With the increased number of fibre-optic handpieces available, it is feasible to have a fibre-optic tip attached to dental units.

Magnification

This is most commonly in the form of magnification loupes, to aid with clinical examination and radiographic evaluation.

Dyes

A variety of different dyes that stain caries are currently available. These help to make the visualisation of caries easier. However, they are primarily used during cavity preparation and result in over preparation and hence are not used routinely.

Radiographic examination

Radiographs can be used to confirm a clinical suspicion of caries, detect early lesions and for monitoring disease activity. Bitewing radiographs are the view of choice for diagnosis of occlusal and proximal caries in posterior teeth; however diagnostic problems may arise because of superimposition of the cuspal pattern and contact point overlap. Periapical radiographs are required for anterior teeth. Extraoral radiographs such as dental panoramic radiographs should not be used for the diagnosis of dental caries owing to their lack of sensitivity[5,6].

Laser fluorescence

Lasers can be used as an aid to detection of caries, especially early enamel lesions. The principle is based on laser fluorescence. Caries illuminated by a laser will fluoresce, the degree to which this occurs is an indicator of the disease process. However, heavy fissure staining can affect the degree of laser fluorescence.

Electrical conduction methods

This principle is based on electrical conductance and the fact that sound enamel is a good electrical insulator; however, carious teeth (with porosities) allow the passage of an electrical current more readily, resulting in a drop in the electrical resistance. The degree to which the resistance drops is an indicator of the extent of caries.

Caries risk assessment

During the initial history, examination and treatment planning for every patient, it is important that there is also an assessment of the patient's individual risk of developing further carious lesions or progression of existing lesions[7]. This procedure is termed *caries risk assessment*. Assuming that all aetiological factors remain equal, this should help in identification of the main causative factors and aid with recommending specific preventive or restorative measures for that individual patient's needs. Dental management of caries may involve operative intervention, but should always incorporate preventive measures. Caries risk assessment carried out during treatment can serve as a monitoring aid for the success of treatment. This assessment should be based upon:

- Caries experience
  - — the extent and number of previous restorations (indicator of past disease)
  - — the extent and number of new lesions
  - — the progression of new lesions.
- Fluoride use – type and frequency.

- Oral hygiene and the extent of plaque present.
- Dietary factors – eating habits, number of main meals, snacks, frequency of fermentable carbohydrate intake.
- Bacterial activity – the presence and amount of cariogenic bacteria, specifically *Lactobacillus* and *Streptococcus mutans*. This may include special laboratory tests.
- Saliva – both the amount (quantity) and buffering capacity (quality).
- Socio-economic status – to evaluate the patient for compliance. Caries tends to be a disease of deprivation and is more prevalent in patients with lower socio-economic status.

The patient's risk of developing further caries can be classified according to the number of caries risk factors present as being high, moderate or low. It is important to bear in mind that a patient's risk assessment can change with time and periodically the assessment of their caries risk should be re-evaluated.

Caries prevention

A decision to intervene in the management of dental caries is probably one of the most important decisions a dentist will make. Early restorative intervention should be avoided if possible as tooth preparation is irreversible and commits the tooth to the restorative cycle[8]. All restorations fail at some time and require either repair/refurbishment or replacement, resulting in yet another insult to the tooth tissues. This repeated insult can ultimately lead to the loss of the tooth. A delayed start on this cycle is advised wherever possible, and there is a resurge in providing early preventive and remineralisation treatment and minimal intervention of carious lesions[8].

Diet

Decreasing the frequency of fermentable carbohydrate consumption and elimination or substitution is essential as this will result in reduced periods of acid production and less risk of demineralisation of the tooth tissue[9].

Fluoride

Fluoride supplements can be either patient or dentist applied. The effects of fluoride on caries in different sites are variable[10]. Fluoride has produced the following reductions in caries:

- 20% in occlusal caries
- 55% in interproximal caries
- 61% in smooth surface caries

It is clear that occlusal caries will still be a significant clinical problem. The topical and systemic effects of fluoride have, however, made the clinical diagnosis of caries more difficult.

Oral hygiene

A well maintained oral hygiene regime helps to maintain the bacterial balance within the oral cavity and can also help to deliver topical fluoride on a regular basis.

MOISTURE CONTROL

The oral cavity is intrinsically a wet environment. The presence of oral fluids (saliva, blood, gingival crevicular fluid and water coolant spray) on the surface of a preparation is likely to:

- Dilute or displace etchant or bonding materials.
- Impair the creation of a bond between tooth and restoration.
- Interfere with cohesion of successive increments of restorative material.
- React with restorative material and thus impair its strength or dimensional stability, e.g. with zinc containing amalgams leading to porosity and expansion.
- Discolour tooth-coloured resin restorations, e.g. with blood contamination.
- Prevent the creation of a marginal seal where a cement lute is employed, e.g. for an indirect restoration.
- Contaminate a site that should preferably have as low a bacterial load as possible, e.g. pulp exposures and root canal therapy.

For these reasons it is necessary to isolate a preparation from moisture, especially when placing restorative materials and undertaking endodontic therapy.

Rubber dam

Rubber dam is the most effective method of moisture control[11–13] and tooth isolation (Fig. 1.10). Rubber dam is available in latex and

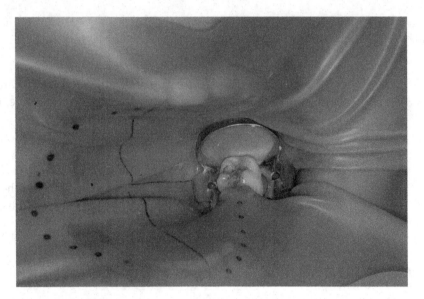

Fig. 1.10 Rubber dam.

latex-free sheets, it can also be obtained in different colours, grades or thickness. Rubber dam has distinct advantages over other methods of moisture control and tooth isolation in that it prevents preparation contamination, protects the airway, aids visibility and reduces the risk of cross infection from patient to operator[14]. The quality of restorations, particularly resin-bonded restorations, is significantly improved by using rubber dam[15]. There is also evidence that patients prefer rubber dam isolation.

It is usual practice, when carrying out restoration placement, to isolate a quadrant or sextant with the tooth under treatment being in the middle. Expertise and experience enhance its convenience. In situations where close application to the cervical margin is difficult, a seal can be obtained by application of a caulking agent or some other sealant, such as light-activated resin.

There are many different techniques for placing and retaining rubber dam. Traditionally, the rubber dam was retained using clamps; however, alternative methods are now available. These include ligatures, such as dental floss or the placement of an alternative interdental retainer such as a portion of rubber dam material, a wooden wedge or commercially available rubber dam retaining aids. If a clamp is used, three different techniques may be employed for placement. These include application of the rubber dam and clamp simultaneously, the rubber dam before the clamp or the clamp before the rubber dam.

Types of clamps for use with rubber dam

A vast array of rubber dam clamps is available, but there are principally four design factors that differ between them. First, and most obvious, is that of size – small clamps are designed to be used on small single-rooted teeth whereas the larger clamps are for use with molar teeth. Clamps are available in a wide variety of sizes reflecting the broad range of sizes of teeth (especially molars) that may be encountered. It is important to realise that if too small a clamp is used then damage to the tooth structure may occur during placement or removal and sensitivity may occur because of pulpal irritation arising from the increased pressure on the tooth with too small a clamp. In addition, if a clamp is too small for a particular tooth, then the bow of the clamp will be stretched to such an extent that fracture of the bow may occur either during, or after, placement. It is for this reason that many clinicians secure one jaw to the other with a floss ligature before application of the dam (though if the floss is left *in situ* after dam placement it may cause leakage).

The jaws of clamps differ in two aspects, namely the presence or absence of 'wings' and the orientation of the jaws. Winged clamps are designed with an extension to the jaws so that the clamp may be positioned into the rubber dam, and clamp and dam applied simultaneously. Winged clamps also have the added advantage that the working area is increased as the wings displace the rubber dam. Wingless clamps do not have extension of the jaws and are placed at a separate stage to the rubber dam, either before or after.

Clamps are retained on the tooth either through engaging the tooth below the maximum bulbosity of the crown, or by actively 'gripping' the tooth surface. The former may be termed bland (or passive) clamps and the jaws have a fairly flat orientation, the latter may be termed 'active' clamps and these often have jaws that are angled gingivally with the points of the jaw closer together than a bland clamp. Active clamps are usually more stable as they are more likely to achieve four-point contact with the tooth. However, the tight fit may cause some post-placement sensitivity and the gingival orientation of the jaws may traumatise the gingivae, as the area of engagement with the tooth is more apical (though this may be an advantage if some gingival retraction is required).

The final design difference relates to clamps that are specifically for retaining rubber dam on anterior teeth while also having the ability to retract the gingivae. These clamps, termed ferrier or butterfly clamps, have a double bow and fine jaws that may be bent to alter the amount

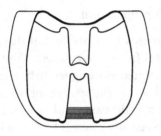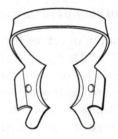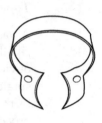

Fig. 1.11 Rubber dam clamps.

of soft tissue retraction that is provided. As the jaws of these clamps are fine, they are not particularly stable and may require support (e.g. with impression compound) to prevent scraping and damaging of the tooth surface.

Thus, clamps for use with rubber dam (Fig. 1.11) may be:

- Various sizes depending on which tooth they are intended for
- Winged or wingless
- Bland or active
- Specifically for anterior teeth and gingival retraction

Other methods of moisture control

Saliva ejector

This may be used routinely during restorative procedures. The flange design is a useful protector and displacer of the tongue when the air turbine is used, it can also be used to reflect light. The saliva ejector is generally held in position by the patient and is therefore dependent on co-operation. It is inadequate on its own, when materials are placed in preparations, but may be supplemented by any of the other moisture control techniques. Cotton wool rolls can be used to stabilise the flange *in situ* and also serve to augment moisture control.

Aspirator

This is a very efficient high volume, low vacuum suction device. It needs continuous chairside assistance for effective operation and therefore cannot be used effectively in single-handed operative dentistry.

Absorbent systems

Cotton wool rolls

These are essential supplements to the saliva ejector during placement of both direct and indirect restorations. They act by absorption and therefore have a limited service life and must be replaced frequently when saturated. The typical requirements for any posterior tooth in a supine patient is three rolls; one in the upper buccal sulcus, one in the lower buccal sulcus and one in the lower lingual sulcus, in order to cope with salivary duct outflow and to collect pooling fluids. Cotton wool rolls are inserted with a rolling action away from the alveolus for stability. In anterior teeth, two rolls are needed in the lower, one buccal and one lingual, while in the upper a minimum of one roll in the upper buccal sulcus. It will be appreciated that rubber dam placement is a more efficient technique.

Cotton wool pellets

These are available in a range of sizes and are useful for drying preparations and cleansing but they have the same limitation of service life and cross infection risk as cotton wool rolls.

Absorbent plaques

These are sheets of absorbent material, which can be adapted to the mucosa, and are arguably more stable than cotton rolls. They have similar limitations of service life but are longer lasting due to the barrier effect.

It is important to note that all absorbents can produce painful after effects, termed cotton burns, if they adhere to dry mucosa and are then forcibly removed. Where such adherence occurs they should be first soaked with water and then gently peeled off.

Air-jet

This is usually applied via an air–water syringe (3-in-1 or triple syringe). It acts merely by forcibly displacing the fluid layer. If applied longer to achieve evaporation effect this technique can result in desiccation of the dentine, which may be injurious to the underlying pulp.

Matrix bands

This is a convenient supplement to other techniques but the coffer dam effect provided by the encircling band can be useful in extreme situations. The band must be well adapted and wedged to be effective in this role.

Pharmacological

This group of agents may have systemic medical implications and are very rarely used in routine practice.

Astringent solutions

These may be applied to control gingival haemorrhage but may cause gingival trauma, if not used with care, as many are caustic or have a low pH.

Adrenaline

One in one thousand adrenaline solution may be applied topically for a short period (up to 2 min) on a cotton pellet to control local gingival bleeding.

Antisialogogues

Antisialogogues, drugs that inhibit oral secretions, appear in all lists of moisture control techniques. However, the use of such drugs is extremely rarely indicated and is generally unsuitable for the ambulant outpatient situation.

Hypnosis

This technique has been suggested for controlling patients' salivary flow rate.

REFERENCES

1. Paul E. A practical guide to assisted operating. 1. Principles of assisted operating. *Br Dent J*, 1972; **133**: 258–61.
2. Paul J.E. Four-handed dentistry. 1. Principles and techniques: a new look. *Dent Update*, 1983; **10**: 155–7, 159–60, 162–4.

3. Kidd E. and Joyston-Bechal S. *Essentials of Dental Caries – The Disease and its Management*, 2nd edn. London, Oxford University Press, 1997.

4. Hicks J., Garcia-Godoy F. and Flaitz C. Biological factors in dental caries enamel structure and the caries process in the dynamic process of demineralization and remineralization (Part 2). *J Clin Pediatr Dent*, 2004; **28**: 119–24.

5. Rushton V.E. and Horner K. The use of panoramic radiology in dental practice. *J Dent*, 1996; **24**: 185–201.

6. Horner K., Rout P.G.J., Rushton V.E. and Wilson N.H.F. *Interpreting Dental Radiographs*. London, Quintessence Publishing, 2002.

7. Reich E., Lussi A. and Newbrun E. Caries-risk assessment. *Int Dent J*, 1999; **49**: 15–26.

8. Anusavice K.J. Management of dental caries as a chronic infectious disease. *J Dent Educ*, 1998; **62**: 791–802.

9. Moynihan P. and Petersen P.E. Diet, nutrition and the prevention of dental diseases. *Public Health Nutr*, 2004; **7**: 201–26.

10. Jacobsen P. and Young D. The use of topical fluoride to prevent or reverse dental caries. *Spec Care in Dent*, 2003; **23**: 177–9.

11. Liebenberg W.H. Extending the use of rubber dam isolation: alternative procedures. Part I. *Quintessence Int*, 1992; **23**: 657–65.

12. Liebenberg W.H. Extending the use of rubber dam isolation: alternative procedures. Part II. *Quintessence Int*, 1993; **24**: 7–17.

13. Liebenberg W.H. Extending the use of rubber dam isolation: alternative procedures. Part III. *Quintessence Int*, 1993; **24**: 237–44.

14. Kidd E.A. Rubber dam – a reappraisal. *Dent Update*, 1983; **10**: 233–40.

15. Christensen G.J. Using rubber dams to boost quality, quantity of restorative services. *J Am Dent Assoc*, 1994; **125**: 81–2.

Principles of
direct intervention

PRESERVATIVE MANAGEMENT

Over recent years the dental profession has shifted towards practising preventive dentistry and adopting more conservative and
tooth-preserving procedures. Such progression is considered to be a
response to the decline in the level of dental caries and increased con-
sumer demands with regards to comfort of treatment and advances in
materials science. This shift in caries management, based on rational
clinical and scientific principles, will no doubt continue over the com-
ing decades[1].

PRINCIPLES OF OPERATIVE INTERVENTION

Modern cavity preparation and design and the evolution thereof
cannot, or perhaps should not, be considered without reference to
G.V. Black. Black's text *A Work on Operative Dentistry* in 1908[2] was the
first to prescribe a systematic method of cavity preparation and the
'ideal' cavity form. These features relate to the instruments available
at the time (slowly rotating burs with poor cutting efficiency and
chisels), caries incidence and pattern, as well as restorative materials
available. Although modifications to the classical cavity forms and
principles to achieve these were suggested in the early 1900s, these
principles remained appropriate and largely unchallenged for a
period of over 50 years. The basic shape, and some of the ideals, of
Black's cavities have been popular until recent times and indeed to a
degree are still prevalent.

The last 35 years have seen tremendous advances in dentistry, in
particular related to tooth-coloured restorative materials and in the

Table 2.1 Black's classification of carious lesions versus current terminology.

Black's classification	Current terminology
Class I	Affecting pits and/or fissures also termed occlusal lesions
Class II	Affecting the proximal surfaces of posterior teeth
Class III	Affecting the proximal surfaces of anterior teeth
Class IV	Affecting the proximal surfaces of anterior teeth and involving the incisal angle
Class V	Affecting the cervical surfaces

bonding of restorative materials to tooth tissue. Such developments have brought about a re-evaluation of Black's principles and, furthermore, a move away from Black's classification of carious lesions and prescribed preparation form. Carious lesions are best described by the site in which they occur and the size of lesion, an approach taken by Mount and Hume[3] in their proposal for a new classification of cavities. Many of the modifications have been made on an empirical basis, with scientific evaluation and suggestions more prevalent in the latter part of the last century (Table 2.1).

In contrast to Black's principles of cavity preparation, which included the establishment of outline form including extension for prevention, the development of resistance and retention form, creation of convenience form, the treatment of residual caries, the finishing of cavity margins and cavity toilet, now the general principles of tooth preparation are determined by:

- The nature and extent of the lesion.
- The quantity and quality of the tooth tissue remaining following preparation.
- Functional load.
- The nature and properties of the restorative system to be used.

In general the minimum amount of tooth substance should be removed to ensure appropriate access and the placement of the required restoration. With developments in the range and properties of the materials available for the restoration of teeth, it is now possible to consider the preparation of teeth as an exercise in damage limitation, with due consideration of both the macroscopic and microscopic features of the biophysical environment into which it is intended to introduce a restoration. This concept was neatly described by

Anusavice[1] as a preservative approach to the operative management of dental caries and associated lesions.

To be able to prepare teeth efficiently and effectively, it is essential to understand the processes of the diseases of teeth, have a detailed working knowledge of tooth anatomy[4], the structure and properties of the tooth tissues and pulp biology, and have a clear understanding of the basic principles of occlusion. In addition, one must understand the mode of action, functions and limitations of the instrumentation used to shape and fashion enamel and dentine in the oral environment.

The process of preparing teeth may be considered to comprise the following stages.

Gaining access

In order to remove caries, create the required form of preparation, and enable restorative materials to be placed, adapted and contoured to restore form and function, it is generally necessary initially to cut through and then cut away part of the enamel of the tooth to be treated. Even when the tooth contains a large lesion, it is generally necessary to gain access using a friction-retained, water-cooled, diamond bur held in an air turbine handpiece. If the lesion to be treated is associated with an existing restoration, the whole restoration may need to be removed using the air-turbine handpiece; however, increasingly the benefits of repairing rather than replacing existing restorations are being acknowledged.

Removal of caries

With access established, caries is removed, first from around the amelodentinal junction and then, working apically, towards the areas overlying the pulp. When caries extends down to a vital pulp, one should aim to remove all soft, stained, infected dentine leaving either some stained but firm dentine or possibly some slightly softened, unstained dentine protecting the pulp from exposure. The rationale for this is that affected dentine (rather than infected dentine) may be retained and remineralised with the use of a therapeutic liner. It is common to experience difficulties in distinguishing between dentine that should be removed, and that which should be left. Fluorescence-aided caries excavation[5] or a caries detector dye have been suggested as aids in such situations, but may actually lead to over-preparation[6]. The area of the amelodentinal junction must always be made completely caries-free, although again the necessity for this has recently been questioned.

Development of final form

Once the caries has been removed, before proceeding to create the final cavity form, it is necessary to consider the biological, functional and mechanical demands that will be placed on the final tooth-restorative 'system'. In particular, the following should be considered.

Minimisation of the effect of preparation on tooth strength

Any preparation will weaken a tooth and predispose it to fracture. To minimise this effect, all internal line angles should be rounded.

Choice of restorative material

The material to be used is dictated largely by the size of the cavity/preparation and an assessment of the functional demands that will be placed on the tooth-restorative system. If the tooth is non-functional then mechanical properties of the material will not be a large consideration, but for a large preparation in a functional tooth a material that is strong (e.g. amalgam) and able to withstand the stresses encountered during function will be required. The choice of material will influence the final form of the preparation, particularly the cavo-surface angle (more critical with amalgam restorations) and presence of retentive features (more required with non-adhesive restorations).

Integrity of the remaining tooth structure

The preparation should be planned to maximise the preservation and protection of remaining tooth structure. Increasing cavity depth and width increases the potential for outward flexion of buccal and lingual walls[7]. Preparations with a curved floor show less cuspal movement than those with a flat floor and a flat floor with its sharp angles and stress concentrations may lead to fracture. This flexure may also have effects on subsequent buccal restorations[8]. If caries has undermined the remaining tooth structure to a significant degree, the tooth may fracture during function. The planned removal of such healthy tissue may, in fact, preserve tooth structure in the long term by minimising the subsequent risk of fracture, which may otherwise lead to loss of a large quantity of strategic tooth structure. Also, it has long been established that there is increased fracture incidence in teeth with restorations of a wide isthmus and having three or more surfaces. The provision of cuspal protection should be considered in such cases.

Placement of margins

Black originally proposed that margins should be placed well into the embrasures in cleansable areas, but the degree to which this has been adopted has slowly reduced over the years with the acceptance that good oral hygiene is sufficient. Cervically, Black recommended that margins should be placed in a caries-free zone subgingivally, but this zone is the area of gingival attachment! It is now accepted that margins should be kept free of the gingivae to avoid periodontal problems and that incidence of overhangs and marginal gaps must be avoided. It may be necessary to extend the preparation if the margin (i.e. interface between tooth structure and restorative material) is close to a contact with an opposing tooth as there is the potential for early breakdown at this weak interface. This emphasises the need to mark the occlusal contacts before preparation is commenced, especially if rubber dam is being used. Similarly, for cavities involving the proximal surface it may be necessary to extend the gingival margin in an apical direction to allow placement of a matrix band. This differs significantly from Black's 'ideal' preparation with predefined placement of margins (Fig. 2.1).

Elderton[9,10] has argued that many amalgam restoration failures are due to marginal breakdown owing to a low amalgam marginal angle (AMA) and high cavo-surface angle (CSA). He has suggested that preparations with AMA of at least 70° (ideally 90°) will yield longer lasting restorations (Fig. 2.2). In a 2-year clinical study of amalgam restorations in preparations with such margins, Stratis and Bryant[11] commented on the difficulty of consistently achieving these angles. They showed that utilising these angles (together with finishing procedures) resulted in fewer marginal fractures although the short-term nature of the study was noted.

Planning of the retentive form

If a non-adhesive restoration is to be placed, some mechanical retention must be included in the preparation. The nature of caries lesions

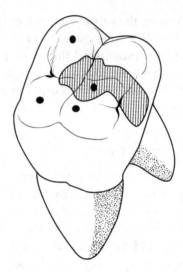

Fig. 2.1 Rounded cavity form and position of occlusal contacts relative to cavity margins.

is such that removal of the caries should result in a preparation that is undercut in cross-section. This general form may provide sufficient retention for the restoration. However, in a large preparation, additional retentive features may need to be provided – these include undercuts, grooves, boxes etc. and these aspects are addressed later in this chapter.

Integrity of the restoration

Internal preparation features affect the stresses that occur within the restoration. This is particularly important in the case of proximal lesions in which the placement of a groove in the floor of the 'box' will minimise the lateral forces to which the restoration is subjected and thus reduce failure due to fracture of the restorative material.

A wide range of rotary and hand instruments may be used to remove unsupported tooth structure and form features within the remaining tooth structure. Such procedures should always be performed in such a way as to minimise pulpal damage. Completed preparations must always be meticulously cleaned, dried and then carefully inspected for evidence of residual caries or small exposures, which may have been overlooked.

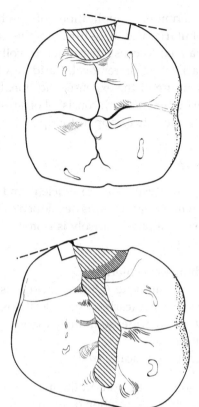

Fig. 2.2 Cavo-surface angle of proximal preparations.

ALTERNATIVE PREPARATION METHODS

Chemomechanical caries removal

Chemomechanical techniques are one of the recently documented alternatives to traditional mechanical rotary techniques and mechanical non-rotary techniques.

Chemomechanical caries removal involves the application of a gel to tooth tissue. This selectively softens the carious dentine, thus facilitating its removal. Removal of sound tooth structure, the cutting of open dentinal tubules, pulpal irritation and pain are all reduced when compared with conventional mechanical methods[12].

The first commercially launched product for chemomechanical caries removal was Caridex (National Patent Medical Products Inc.), initially introduced on the US market in 1985. This system involved the intermittent application of preheated N-monochloro-DL-2-aminobutyric acid (GK-101E) to the carious lesion. The solution was claimed to cause disruption of collagen in the carious dentine, thus facilitating its removal. Caridex was not widely adopted, possibly because of the expense, additional clinical time and the bulky delivery system, which consisted of a reservoir, a heater, a pump and a handpiece with an applicator tip.

Carisolv

During the 1990s a more efficient and effective chemomechanical caries removal system was developed called Carisolv™ (Medi Team). The formulation of Carisolv is isotonic in nature and consists of the following:

- Sodium hypochlorite (0.5%)
- Three amino acids (glutamic acid, leusine, lysine)
- Gel substance (carboxymethylcellulose)
- Sodium chloride/sodium hydroxide
- Saline solution
- Colouring indicator (red)

Carisolv can be used in the management of the majority of caries lesions, either in isolation or in conjunction with a handpiece, which may be required to gain access or remove existing restorations. The clinical situations in which Carisolv could be considered the preferred method of caries removal include:

- When the preservation of tooth structure is important (this should be every case).
- The removal of root/cervical caries, where access and visibility are good.
- The management of coronal caries with cavitation, thus avoiding the use of dental handpieces.
- The removal of caries at the margins of crowns and bridge abutments, thus decreasing the likelihood of replacing the entire crown/bridge.
- The completion of tunnel preparations (where access to approximal caries is gained via the occlusal surface, leaving the marginal ridge intact).
- Ensuring complete caries removal.
- Where local anaesthesia is contraindicated.
- The care of caries in dentally anxious patients (needle phobics).

- Management of primary carious lesions in deciduous teeth.
- Atraumatic restorative technique (ART) procedures.
- Caries management in special needs patients.

The last five situations should result in the avoidance of local anaesthetic administration.

The clinical technique employed can be quickly and easily mastered. However, careful case selection is initially required. For the first few cases, it is advisable to select fully visible and easily accessible lesions such as buccal root caries or occlusal caries with 1–2 mm entry opening, thus allowing the procedure to be observed. Early cavitation usually helps to provide easy access for gel application and instrumentation, and does not necessitate the use of a handpiece to gain access. From a patient perspective the response to the technique has been almost universally positive, with patients reporting less pain, discomfort and shorter perceived treatment times when compared with traditional drilling[13]. The avoidance of both slow-speed cutting and, in many cases, the use of a high-speed handpiece, makes the experience relatively pleasant for the patient. However in some instances, it is still necessary to use the high-speed handpiece with water coolant to gain access.

A number of theories have been postulated as to why there may be reduced pain and need for local anaesthesia. These include the lack of cutting into caries-free dentine, relatively few dentine tubules are exposed, no vibrations from drilling, no great temperature variations and the dentine is constantly covered with an isotonic gel at body temperature. The possible psychological input of a quiet and less traumatic experience may also play an important role. In certain cases it is necessary to administer a local anaesthetic to complete deep cavity preparation or where existing restorations, crown and bridgework require removal before cavity preparation.

Sonic preparation

Sonic instruments have been used within the field of dentistry for many decades, principally for scaling and root surface debridement. Their use for cavity preparation has been revisited recently. The system was initially marketed for proximal lesions with matching size preparation tips and ceramic inserts. This type of approach proved to be destructive to the tooth tissue. The newer sonic handpieces allow for interchangeable tips and multiple applications, such as minimally invasive caries therapy, cavity preparations, endodontics, periodontics, luting procedures and prophylaxis.

Air abrasion

Air abrasion has also been revisited in recent years in light of developments in restorative materials and changes in cavity preparation design. Most units work by delivery of a jet of aluminium oxide particles at a pressure of 40–149 psi (276–1028 kPa) through a fine nozzle. It is these spray particles that effectively cut the tooth tissue and restorative materials. Air abrasion is best suited to the treatment of small lesions in pits and fissures, cervical caries and recurrent caries around existing restorations. The advantages of such a system include: a local anaesthetic is usually not required; several lesions in different quadrants can be completed at one visit; saucer-shaped preparations can be produced and these are ideal for resin-bonded restorations; and there is less noise and vibration compared with the slow handpiece. However, over-spray can contaminate the surgery, clog the handpiece bearings, block the suction units and damage unprotected adjacent teeth. It is claimed that newer air abrasion units eliminate these problems with high volume suction and water to reduce the over-spray. This method is not very effective for removal of soft caries, therefore manual excavation or slow handpiece removal is required. Some practitioners use chemomechanical caries removal in conjunction with air abrasion. Air abrasion cannot be used for precise cavity preparations, such as inlays or crowns.

Lasers

The field of laser technology has developed considerably over recent years, and many types of lasers are available for cutting of dental hard tissue. The combined CO_2/erbium substituted: yttrium aluminium garnet (Er:YAG) dental laser is designed for cutting both hard and soft tissue. It has been reported to be as fast as a turbine handpiece, silent and does not require the use of a local anaesthetic for the preparation of enamel and dentine. Their use for soft-tissue surgery has been well documented; however there is limited literature available on dental hard tissue and some concern has been raised about heat generation.

PULP PROTECTION

In discussing aspects of pulp protection, it is useful to consider definitions of a sealer, liner and base[14]:

- *Sealer* – a cavity sealer is a material which seals the dentinal tubules and provides a protective coating for the freshly cut tooth structure of the prepared cavity.
- *Liner* – a cavity liner is an aqueous or volatile organic suspension or dispersion of zinc oxide or calcium hydroxide that can be applied to a cavity surface in a relatively thin film. Glass-ionomer cement and resin-modified glass-ionomer cements are also suitable for use as lining materials.
- *Base* – a cavity base is a material, usually a type of cement, used to base a prepared cavity before the insertion of a permanent restoration, to protect the pulp and act as a dentine replacement.

Historical concepts

Microleakage is the term used for the passing of fluids, micro-organisms or ions between the restoration and the adjacent preparation walls. Microleakage occurs around all restorations currently used in restorative dentistry, including those that are adhesively bonded to enamel and dentine. Such leakage provides a path for the ingress of bacteria and their products around restorations and has been implicated in a variety of clinical conditions, including marginal discoloration, pulpal irritation and subsequent necrosis, postoperative sensitivity, recurrent caries and eventual failure of restorations[15,16].

The methods used to treat the preparation walls before restoration placement have changed over the years. This is thought to be a response to better understanding of the cause of pulpal damage, Brannstrom's hydrodynamic theory of pulpal pain[17,18] and the development of new dental materials.

Traditional dental teaching advocated the generous use of bases and liners under restorations (especially amalgam) to limit postoperative sensitivity and to act as a thermal insulator. It was originally thought that the primary cause of pulpal inflammation was related to the direct cytotoxic effect of the dental restorative material. However, this has been shown to be a mild and transitory effect[18].

Current concepts

Most authorities now recognise that the presence of bacteria is the most important determinant factor of pulp inflammation and ultimately pulp death. Bacterial contamination may be derived from the initial carious lesion, cavity preparation and restoration placement, the smear layer or microleakage. Hilton[14] stated that 'an understanding of the properties of the currently available materials, and how they interact with the pulpal tissue, can help the practitioner decide when to use bases and liners and which products to choose.' The routine placement of a preparation liner or base is now not advocated. All preparations should have some form of preparation sealer and some preparations (usually deep) will require a liner and/or base.

The pulp may be damaged during the restorative procedure by inadequate water cooling of the burs, use of worn burs or by accidental entry into the pulp chamber (pulpal exposure) by hand or rotary instruments. Accurate knowledge of the anatomy of each tooth is therefore essential to ensure that tooth preparation is completed with the minimum of iatrogenic damage. An important consideration here is the age of the patient, in that younger patients have larger pulp chambers than older patients.

To prevent further noxious stimuli reaching the pulp it has been usual practice to protect further the pulp by applying therapeutic materials to the floor and/or the pulpo-axial wall of the preparation. These materials were commonly placed under amalgams and resin composites to prevent thermal stimulation of the pulp and acid contamination of dentine respectively. It has now been demonstrated that thermal stimulation of dentine is not a problem clinically and that routine basing of amalgams, to prevent thermal stimulation, inherently weakens the restoration. It is also now accepted that dentine can be etched and therefore routine lining for resin composites is now contraindicated.

Sealer

Traditionally, cavity varnishes have been routinely used to provide a protective coating for freshly cut tooth structure. A cavity varnish is a natural gum, such as copal or rosin, or a synthetic resin dissolved in an organic solvent such as acetone, chloroform or ether, which evaporates and leaves a protective film behind. Many studies support the view that the application of a cavity varnish under amalgam restorations provides a temporary seal, decreasing microleakage until corrosion products are deposited. Doubts have been expressed as to the effectiveness of Copalite varnish to seal teeth restored with high copper amalgam long enough for corrosion products to be deposited at the interface[19]. The increased microleakage seen with some high copper amalgam restorations may be due to the fact that the varnish dissolves before the corrosion products are fully formed. Recent advances in dentine bonding agents have led to recommendations for their use under amalgam restorations to seal the dentinal tubules, eliminate dentinal fluid movement, decrease microleakage and post-operative temperature sensitivity.

In recent years various desensitising agents have been used in the management of tooth hypersensitivity. These agents are reported to be effective by reducing the diameter of the dentinal tubule and limiting fluid movement[20]. It has been postulated that the application of the same mechanism allows desensitising agents to be equally effective in preventing postoperative sensitivity when amalgam restorations are placed. These materials may be of value in the treatment of cavity surfaces before amalgam placement.

Liner

Cavity liners are placed to a thickness of typically less than 0.5 mm. They act as cavity sealers and may have the additional therapeutic benefits of fluoride release, adhesion to tooth structure and antibacterial properties. Liners may not have sufficient thickness or strength to be used alone in deep preparations; therefore they are frequently overlaid by a base material. The most popular currently used cavity liners are calcium hydroxide and glass-ionomer cements. Resin-modified light-activated glass-ionomer liner materials have gained increased popularity and have the added advantage of ease of placement, command set and early resistance to moisture contamination. Eugenol based materials are contraindicated as liners for resin composite restorations, because the eugenol may be absorbed into the resin composite, act as a plasticiser and decrease bond strength. This view has, however, been disputed over recent years[21,22].

Base

The ideal base material is a thermal insulator, non-toxic, cariostatic, has persistent antibacterial properties, is able to stimulate reparative dentine formation, and is strong enough to withstand the forces of amalgam condensation and masticatory forces. Bases are traditionally dentine replacement materials, and may also be used to block out undercuts for indirect restorations. All cement bases dissolve slowly and disintegrate with time in the oral environment. They act as a mechanical barrier between the restorative material and the underlying pulp. The remaining dentine thickness overlying the pulp is the single most important factor when deciding whether or not to place a base. In vitro studies have shown that a remaining dentine thickness of between 0.5 and 1 mm reduces the toxicity levels of materials by 75% and 90% respectively[23]. Dentine is said to be the most effective base and should not be removed to accommodate a proprietary material.

The most commonly used bases have been zinc polycarboxylate, glass-ionomer cements, zinc oxide eugenol and zinc phosphate cements.

On the basis of research, the philosophy of basing a preparation to an ideal form has fallen into disrepute. Bases have few benefits and make the restoration more prone to fracture. The main question today has to be whether cement bases under amalgam restorations are necessary and have any value in current operative dentistry techniques.

Materials that are used for bases can sometimes be used for temporary dressings. If a patient has lost a restoration or when tooth preparation is not completed, it is usual to insert a temporary restorative material (temporary dressing). This is designed to seal the preparation and prevent pain from exposed tooth substance and to preclude further carious activity until a permanent restoration can be placed.

Indications for use

Dentine itself is an excellent insulator; therefore, in preparations estimated to have more than 2 mm of remaining dentine thickness, there is generally no requirement for any pulp protective material beneath the restorative material. However a preparation sealer should be placed to seal dentinal tubules and thus prevent post-operative sensitivity and bacterial contamination of dentinal tubules. In the case of simple amalgam restorations two coats of a dentine desensitiser (such as a HEMA/glutardialdehyde combination, available as a proprietary product) may be used. Current research would seem to suggest that cavity varnish will be replaced by dentine bonding agents in the near future. However, there is insufficient evidence, at present, to support the routine use of dentine bonding agents under amalgam restorations. There is growing evidence that compound or complex amalgams would benefit from the application of a dentine bonding agent. Dentine bonding agents should be used routinely used under all resin composite restorations.

For deeper cavities in which there is less than 2 mm of remaining dentine a preparation liner should be placed in the deepest aspects of the preparation. Traditionally, calcium hydroxide was used routinely as a liner but is now reserved for use in deeper cavities or for 'capping' procedures (Fig. 2.3).

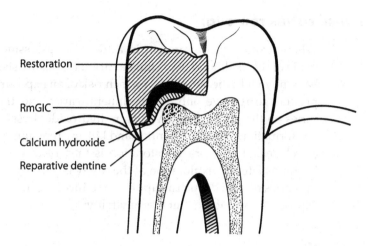

Fig. 2.3 Features of a restored deep lesion (RmGIC = resin-modified glass-ionomer cement).

Table 2.2 Amalgam and resin composite restoration preparation.

	Minimum (just into dentine)	**Moderate** (**more** than 2 mm of dentine remaining)	**Deep** (**less** than 2 mm of dentine remaining)
Amalgam restoration	(S) with dentine desensitiser	(L) with glass-ionomer cement *and* (S) with dentine desensitiser	(L) with glass-ionomer cement always *and* (S) with dentine desensitiser. Hard setting calcium hydroxide may be placed in deeper areas if indicated
Resin composite restoration	(S) with dentine bonding agent	(S) with dentine bonding agent	(L) with calcium hydroxide and glass-ionomer cement in deeper areas if indicated *and* (S) with dentine bonding agent

(S) = Sealer; (L) = Liner; (B) = Base.

Table 2.2 provides a guide to the use of pulp protection materials, indicating suitable combinations of sealers, liners and bases to be used in resin composite and amalgam preparations.

Stepwise caries removal

Where gross caries is present in a tooth, an assessment should be made of the likelihood of creating a carious exposure should all caries be removed. In the situation in which risk of an exposure is high, it is prudent to remove only the peripheral caries and the majority of caries on the pulpal floor. A calcium hydroxide dressing (to encourage formation of tertiary dentine and kill any remaining bacteria) and a well-sealed temporary restoration is then placed. Approximately 3 months later, re-exploration of the cavity is performed and remaining caries removed. Such an approach reduces the incidence of pulpal exposures and subsequent loss of vitality[24,25].

Pulp capping

Direct pulp capping

A direct pulp cap is the term for the procedure in which a dressing/lining (or restorative material) is placed into direct contact with exposed pulpal tissue. This is usually carried out following a carious or traumatic exposure. Calcium hydroxide is most commonly used; however some workers have directly bonded resin composite over exposures and mineral trioxide aggregate may show promise as an alternative (although currently it is relatively expensive).

Indirect pulp capping

An indirect pulp cap is essentially where not all carious affected dentine has been removed and involves placement of a dressing on the deepest dentine. There is some confusion in the literature (even in recent publications) with regards to definition of 'indirect pulp cap'. This term is often used to describe the situation where stained, demineralised dentine is not removed and a calcium hydroxide lining placed to encourage formation of tertiary dentine and kill any remaining bacteria. An alternative definition is where calcium hydroxide is used in a similar manner over soft, carious dentine.

Greater understanding of the caries process has led to the distinction between infected and affected dentine[26]. Stained dentine may be affected by caries (may be slightly demineralised or conversely may be sclerosed) but may not necessarily be infected and thus removal of such dentine would, in fact, be over preparation with unnecessary loss of tooth structure. Thus it could be argued that the first definition of an indirect pulp cap (where stained, demineralised dentine is not removed and a calcium hydroxide lining placed) reflects nothing more than routine practice for pulp protection.

Although several studies have been completed with regard to progression of caries and prognosis of teeth in which permanent restorations are placed over caries, there is at present insufficient evidence to support this approach. Thus the second approach to indirect pulp capping (where soft, carious dentine is left) describes a procedure that, with current evidence, should not be performed.

Given the above arguments and with confusion over the term indirect pulp cap, it is best to avoid this term and consider the use of calcium hydroxide for three lining purposes:

- For *deeper cavities* where it is estimated that less than 2 mm of dentine remains, a preparation liner should be placed in the deepest parts of the preparation (to encourage formation of tertiary dentine and minimise risk of future exposure).
- For *direct pulp capping* procedures (to stimulate formation of calcific repair).
- For *stepwise caries removal* (to encourage formation of tertiary dentine, kill any remaining bacteria and reduce risk of exposure).

SUPPLEMENTARY RETENTION FOR DIRECT RESTORATIONS

Retention is the ability of a restoration to resist forces that would dislodge it in the long axis of the tooth. Resistance of a restoration is the ability of a restoration to resist forces that would dislodge it in a lateral or rotational direction. In general terms, features of a preparation that provide resistance form will also provide some degree of retention, and the two terms are often interchanged.

Retention of a restoration within the tooth relies primarily on there being sufficient coronal tooth tissue which can provide:

- Adequate bulk of dentine to form an undercut preparation or allow for placement of undercuts without resulting in weakened tooth structure.
- Sufficient coronal tooth tissue to provide 'bracing' to lateral forces and hence provide some resistance to displacement of the restoration.

Often with extensively broken down teeth it is impossible to develop appropriate retention and resistance form with the remaining tooth tissues and alternative methods to retain the restoration must be considered. A variety of techniques may be employed (perhaps in combination) to provide the extra retention.

Bonding

The principle of acid etching of enamel and the use of resin-based adhesives with resin composite materials is well established and the continuing development of multi-purpose bonding systems has allowed such materials to be bonded to tooth structure in a broad range of situations without the need to sacrifice healthy tooth structure in order to increase retention and resistance. A more difficult situation arises when the material being used does not bond to tooth structure. Retention is normally provided by undercuts and preparation features; however at times it may not be possible to create these features. This is classically the case with amalgam restorations in large preparations. With any operative procedure, there is a fundamental need to preserve tooth structure wherever possible and this equally applies to situations in which additional retention is required. In this respect, the ability to achieve additional retention through bonding restorative materials to tooth structure (and rely less on mechanical means of resistance) offers obvious advantages.

A variety of propriety adhesives that are specifically for use in bonding amalgam to tooth structure are now available[27]. These are principally bi-functional polymeric resins, for example phosphonated esters of bis-GMA, 4-META and HEMA. Most of these adhesives bond to enamel and dentine in a similar way to resin composite bonding systems, though the bond between amalgam and adhesive is thought to be purely micromechanical[28].

Numerous *in vitro* studies related to bonded amalgam restorations have been reported in the literature. Despite there being few long-term clinical studies, there are definite short-term advantages, including: preservation of tooth structure, decreased immediate postoperative sensitivity, increased retention and increased fracture resistance of remaining tooth structure[29–31]. The long-term benefits are, however, less certain, reflecting uncertainty regarding the durability of the resin bond. In addition it should not be forgotten that bonding an amalgam restoration requires a well-controlled operating field and may be more time consuming.

When the short-term benefits of bonding amalgam restorations are of use, for example to reinforce weakened cusps before providing a cuspal coverage restoration (large cores, or endodontically treated teeth), there seems little excuse for not adopting such a procedure. The long-term benefit of bonding amalgam restorations is uncertain. Therefore, given the lack of long-term clinical data, increased cost and technique sensitivity, the use of adhesive liners under amalgam restorations cannot yet be advocated as a routine procedure.

Preparation design features

In general, once carious dentine has been removed from a cavity, the resulting shape will be undercut; however this general shape may not be sufficient to retain a restoration when the preparation/restoration is particularly large. In order to increase the retention and resistance form of a preparation, the placement of well-defined preparation features such as undercuts, slots and grooves will often suffice (Fig. 2.4). These include parallelism or relative undercuts of all preparation walls, proximal box form, retention grooves in the proximal line angles and box form in buccal and lingual groove areas of molars. Although healthy tooth structure should be retained whenever possible, the careful and judicious removal of dentine to create retentive features will result in enhanced service of the restoration and ultimately greater longevity of the tooth itself due to fewer interventions over the lifespan of the tooth. Defined preparation features can be easily and safely cut into remaining dentine with a variety of small burs. In order for these features to have maximum benefit, they should be placed in opposing dentine walls.

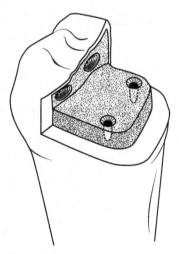

Fig. 2.4 Supplementary features for retention of direct restorations.

In a large preparation with one or more missing cusps, the resulting preparation floor is often fairly flat in its entire profile. If this preparation were filled with no additional preparation features, even when there are significant undercuts in the remaining dentine walls, the ability of the restoration to withstand lateral forces will be limited. The placement of a circumferential groove or shelf will provide a significant increase in the resistance form of the preparation.

The preparation of circular chambers cut vertically into dentine of about 1–1.5 mm diameter and 2 mm deep, into which restorative material is placed, can provide resistance and retention. These features have also been termed amalgam inserts or amalgapins.

A disadvantage of slot-retained amalgam restorations is that they are particularly sensitive to displacement during matrix removal, and great care must be taken not to dislodge the restoration when removing the matrix.

Dentine pins

The use of dentine pins is well established as a method of providing additional retention (Fig. 2.5). Three types of pin (cemented, friction-

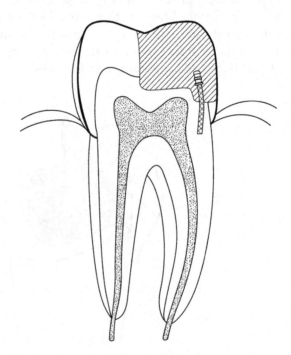

Fig. 2.5 Typical position of a dentine pin.

locked and self-threading) have been used to retain dental restorations. Although cemented and friction-locked pins have certain advantages, all but a few of the pins presently used in clinical practice are of the self-threading type. These are relatively simple to use and are the most retentive. A wide variety of self-threading pins are available, a typical dentine pin system comprises a twist drill with a matching pin, which is usually threaded and self-tapping (i.e. cuts its own thread on insertion). It is usual that both drill and pin have a latch grip enabling them to be used in a conventional handpiece. Some pins consist of a simple length of threaded pin, while others have features such as a shoulder stop (to control depth of insertion) and altered shapes for more mechanical retention of the restorative material.

Although the use of dentine pins has an advantage over preparation features in that less removal of sound tooth structure is required, it has long been recognised that their use also has considerable problems. The stress produced within the dentine during placement of a dentine pin causes cracking and subsequent weakening. Errors during placement are not uncommon and may result in perforations into the pulpal space or the periodontal ligament with subsequent problems. An additional problem may occur due to the mismatch of the modulus of elasticity of the pin and the restorative material. This, combined with the lack of homogeneity of the restorative material due to pin placement, may cause localised stress concentrations during load and a subsequent predisposition to failure (i.e. pins weaken rather than reinforce or strengthen restorations). This can be a problem with amalgam and more so with polymeric restorative materials where such a mismatch will be even larger. Obviously, the more pins that are placed, the greater the risks.

Given the routine use of bonding agents with polymeric restorative materials, the additional use of dentine pins with these materials is questionable as the disadvantages would seem to outweigh any advantages. In addition if an adhesively retained restoration is supplemented with dentine pin placement, catastrophic bond failure may go unnoticed and rapidly progressing caries is then a risk.

There is a lack of clinical data on survival of large amalgam restorations placed with or without pin retention[32,33]. There are however, some studies that suggest that large amalgam restorations placed without the use of dentine pins, but using preparation features as described above have equal strength, resistance and longevity to those restorations placed with pin retention. It is becoming apparent that supplementary retention/resistance is probably not as essential as was once thought, and when necessary can be achieved without the use of dentine pins and their potential problems. For very large restorations, the placement of a dentine pin can aid in stabilising the amalgam during removal of the matrix band and during finishing. In this way dentine pins may be useful for a particularly large amalgam restoration that is otherwise retained by preparation features as described above.

Amalgam dowel core

An amalgam dowel core, also termed a Nayyar core (after the clinician who first reported the technique), is a method described for restoration of endodontically treated molars before provision of an indirect restoration such as a crown[34]. This direct core utilises the coronal pulp space and a few millimetres of the radicular canal for retention. This corono-radicular core (Nayyar core) is described fully in Chapter 4.

REFERENCES

1. Anusavice K.J. Management of dental caries as a chronic infectious disease. *J Dent Educ*, 1998; **62**: 791–802.
2. Black G.V. *A Work on Operative Dentistry*. London, Claudius Ash, 1908.
3. Mount G.J. and Hume W.R. A new cavity classification. *Aust Dent J*, 1998; **43**: 153–9.
4. Van Beek G.C. *Dental Morphology: An Illustrated Guide*, 2nd edn. Bristol, Wright, 1983.
5. Lennon A.M. Fluorescence-aided caries excavation (FACE) compared to conventional method. *Oper Dent*, 2003; **28**: 341–5.
6. Banerjee A., Kidd E.A. and Watson T.F. *In vitro* validation of carious dentin removed using different excavation criteria. *Am J Dent*, 2003; **16**: 228–30.
7. Granath L. and Svensson A. Elastic outward bending of loaded buccal and lingual premolar walls in relation to cavity size and form. *Scand J Dent Res*, 1991; **99**: 1–7.
8. Rees J.S. and Jacobsen P.H. The effect of cuspal flexure on a buccal Class V restoration: a finite element study. *J Dent*, 1998; **26**: 361–7.
9. Elderton R.J. Restorations without conventional cavity preparations. *Int Dent J*, 1988; **38**: 112–8.
10. Elderton R.J. Cavo-surface angles, amalgam margin angles and occlusal cavity preparations. *Br Dent J*, 1984; **156**: 319–24.
11. Stratis S. and Bryant R.W. The influence of modified cavity design and finishing techniques on the clinical performance of amalgam restorations: a 2-year clinical study. *J Oral Rehabil*, 1998; **25**: 269–78.

12. Morrow L.A., Hassall D.C., Watts D.C. and Wilson N.H.F. A chemome-chanical method for caries removal. *Dent Update*, 2000; **27**: 398–401.

13. Anusavice K.J. and Kincheloe J.E. Comparison of pain associated with mechanical and chemomechanical removal of caries. *J Dent Res*, 1987; **66**: 1680–3.

14. Hilton T.J. Cavity sealers, liners, and bases: current philosophies and indications for use. *Oper Dent*, 1996; **21**: 134–46.

15. Bergenholtz G., Cox C.F., Loesche W.J. and Syed S.A. Bacterial leakage around dental restorations: its effect on the dental pulp. *J Oral Pathol*, 1982; **11**: 439–50.

16. Going R.E. Microleakage around dental restorations: a summarizing review. *J Am Dent Assoc*, 1972; **84**: 1349–57.

17. Brannstrom M., Linden L.A. and Astrom A. The hydrodynamics of the dental tubule and of pulp fluid. A discussion of its significance in relation to dentinal sensitivity. *Caries Res*, 1967; **1**: 310–7.

18. Brannstrom M. The cause of postrestorative sensitivity and its pre-vention. *J Endod*, 1986; **12**: 475–81.

19. Fitchie J.G., Reeves G.W., Scarbrough A.R. and Hembree J.H. Microleak-age of a new cavity varnish with a high-copper spherical amalgam alloy. *Oper Dent*, 1990; **15**: 136–40.

20. Trowbridge H.O. and Silver D.R. A review of current approaches to in-office management of tooth hypersensitivity. *Dent Clin North Am*, 1990; **34**: 561–81.

21. Peutzfeldt A. and Asmussen E. Influence of eugenol-containing tem-porary cement on efficacy of dentin-bonding systems. *Eur J Oral Sci*, 1999; **107**: 65–9.

22. Ganss C. and Jung M. Effect of eugenol-containing temporary cements on bond strength of composite to dentin. *Oper Dent*, 1998; **23**: 55–62.

23. Meryon S.D. An *in vitro* study of factors contributing to the blandness of zinc oxide-eugenol preparations *in vivo*. *Int Endod J*, 1988; **21**: 200–4.

24. Leksell E., Ridell K., Cvek M. and Mejare I. Pulp exposure after stepwise versus direct complete excavation of deep carious lesions in young posterior permanent teeth. *Endod Dent Traumatol*, 1996; **12**: 192–6.

25. Smith A.J., Murray P.E. and Lumley P.J. Preserving the vital pulp in operative dentistry: I. A biological approach. *Dent Update*, 2002; **29**: 64–9.

26. Banerjee A., Watson T.F. and Kidd E.A. Dentine caries: take it or leave it? *Dent Update*, 2000; **27**: 272–6.

27. Setcos J.C., Staninec M. and Wilson N.H.F. The development of resin-bonding for amalgam restorations. *Br Dent J*, 1999; **186**: 328–32.

28. Geiger S.B., Mazor Y., Klein E. and Judes H. Characterization of dentin-bonding-amalgam interfaces. *Oper Dent*, 2001; **26**: 239–47.

29. Hansen E.K. and Asmussen E. *In vivo* fractures of endodontically treated posterior teeth restored with enamel-bonded resin. *Endod Dent Traumatol*, 1990; **6**: 218–25.

30. Mach Z., Regent J., Staninec M., Mrklas L. and Setcos J.C. The integrity of bonded amalgam restorations: a clinical evaluation after five years. *J Am Dent Assoc*, 2002; **133**: 460–7.

31. Summitt J.B., Burgess J.O., Berry T.G., *et al*. The performance of bonded vs. pin-retained complex amalgam restorations: a five-year clinical evaluation. *J Am Dent Assoc*, 2001; **132**: 923–31.

32. Smales R.J. Longevity of cusp-covered amalgams: survivals after 15 years. *Oper Dent*, 1991; **16**: 17–20.

33. Plasmans P.J., Creugers N.H. and Mulder J. Long-term survival of extensive amalgam restorations. *J Dent Res*, 1998; **77**: 453–60.

34. Nayyar A., Walton R.E. and Leonard L.A. An amalgam coronal-radicular dowel and core technique for endodontically treated posterior teeth. *J Prosthet Dent*, 1980; **43**: 511–5.

Principles of endodontics

3

INTRODUCTION

Endodontology is related to processes that take place in, or originate from, contents of the pulpal chamber. Under normal conditions, the pulp is protected by the hard tissues of the tooth and an intact periodontium. Kakehashi *et al.*[1] showed that when the dental pulps in germ-free rats were exposed, reactionary dentine was formed. However, surgical exposure of teeth in rats kept in a conventional microbial environment resulted in the development of pulpal necrosis and apical periodontitis. Therefore, micro-organisms (such as those associated with the caries process) and their by-products may gain access to the pulp and stimulate an inflammatory response. The pulp may maintain its function, but continued stimulation will result in its irreversible destruction and complete breakdown. A necrotic pulp does not have a defence mechanism, and the enclosed environment of the pulp chamber is a favourable medium in which anaerobic bacteria may proliferate. This inflammatory process may then spread beyond the confines of the pulp chamber and into the periapical tissues with consequent tissue damage and resorption of periapical bone. Early signs may be seen on a radiograph as loss of apical lamina dura, more extensive destruction of the periapical tissues may result in stimulation of epithelial cells in the apical region, which can then cause formation of a cyst.

Therefore, treatment of the irreversibly damaged or necrotic pulp should be by removal of the damaged tissue and its replacement with a root filling, the overall aim being to control the intra-canal infection. The canal system is cleaned with files and antimicrobial irrigating solutions before being filled with an inert material (root filling) to prevent further microbial ingress. It is also necessary to have excellent moisture control, so that the canal system can be dried when required, and also to ensure that contamination of the canal system with salivary bacteria does not occur: airway protection is also required owing to the risk of dropping the small instruments. To achieve these objectives, placement of a rubber dam is essential.

The response to endodontic treatment is measured in terms of clinical signs and symptoms and radiographic evidence of healing. If healing is not satisfactory it is necessary to make a decision as to whether the tooth should be re-treated, treated via a surgical approach or extracted.

DIAGNOSIS AND ASSESSMENT

A problem in endodontics is that both the healthy and the damaged pulp are in an enclosed environment (the pulp chamber), hence cannot be directly subjected to diagnostic testing. A further complicating factor is that pain is notoriously subjective and if severe, it may be difficult to identify the causative tooth with certainty. More than one tooth may be involved, so it is essential that the clinical signs and symptoms and the diagnostic tests and radiographs are interpreted carefully and related to the provisional diagnosis.

In determining endodontic requirements, the clinician must decide whether or not there is any pulpal or periapical pathology. This means differentiating between those teeth that are normal, reversibly inflamed, irreversibly inflamed and necrotic. Periapically, it must be determined whether teeth are normal, root treated and normal, or have apical pathology.

Clinical manifestations

The most common clinical manifestation of pulp disease is that of pain. The nature and duration of pain is related to the type and stage of the disease process and may vary from a transient discomfort to throbbing incessant pain. Other diagnostic signs include extra-oral swelling, intra-oral swelling, sinus formation, tooth mobility, periodontal pocketing, tooth discoloration, tooth fracture and caries.

Assessment of pulp vitality

It is understood that in a non-vital tooth there is an absence of both neural and vascular supplies. However, almost all conventional pulp tests employ assessment of the neural supply.

Endodontic treatment should not be undertaken on the basis of pulpal status alone. The patient's medical history, the overall treatment plan and the periodontal status must also be taken into consideration. There are also contraindications to endodontics. These may be divided into general aspects such as factors in the medical history of relevance, poor access, poor oral hygiene and local factors, for example the tooth being unrestorable, the periodontal support being poor, the presence of advanced resorptive defects and complex root morphology.

Electronic testers

In the past, these have been of limited value due to the high incidence of false readings. The latest testers, however, appear to be promising but their use is limited if full coverage restorations are in place. Pulp testers stimulate neural tissue, and there is not necessarily a direct correlation between the existence of nervous tissue and a viable blood flow. Additionally, patients' pain thresholds vary. The actual reading is not important, as it cannot measure any degree of degeneration. However, testing contralateral teeth can give the clinician an indication of pulpal involvement.

Thermal tests

Cold is the more useful test as it is safer and uses a constant temperature. The use of a cotton pellet soaked in a volatile liquid (for example ethyl chloride) is a common method, though sticks of ice may also be used. Although heat is not routinely used, it is helpful when the only symptom is that of heat sensitivity and the patient cannot identify the tooth. Heat may be applied with a warm stick of gutta-percha, though care must be taken to lubricate the tooth surface to be tested with petroleum jelly to prevent the hot gutta-percha from sticking to the tooth and possibly causing a thermal injury. Another method of applying heat is to isolate an individual tooth with rubber dam and syringe hot water over the tooth.

Percussion

The most reliable indication of significant periapical inflammation is that of tenderness to percussion. Periodontal inflammation, which produces milder symptoms, can be identified by finger pressure applied to the tooth in question.

Selective analgesia

This test has gained popularity in recent years, but is generally more effective in localising affected areas rather than individual teeth.

Transillumination

This method is useful in the diagnosis of vertical crown fractures.

Radiography

Radiographic examination is a useful and necessary diagnostic aid. However, it must be remembered that pathology does not result in immediate radiographic changes and periapical changes are not usually seen until the cortical plate within the socket becomes involved (seen radiographically as a loss of definition of the lamina dura). It may be necessary to take more than one radiograph at different angles. Good quality radiographs, a paralleling technique and proper film development are essential for accurate diagnosis.

ENDODONTIC IMAGING

Endodontic radiology utilises periapical radiographs[2]. Diagnosis, treatment and follow-up radiographs for endodontic treatment are preferably taken by the paralleling technique using special film holders.

Preliminary radiographs

A preliminary radiograph of the tooth is necessary before endodontic treatment[3]. There must be minimal distortion of the final image; a paralleling technique and film holder should be used. Any pre-existing radiographs of the tooth should be consulted as they may contribute useful information about progression of a periapical lesion and anatomy of the tooth and neighbouring structures.

Ideally, a periapical radiograph should cover the full length of the tooth root(s) and at least 2 mm of periapical bone. Should there be evidence of a periapical radiolucency the area of the entire lesion and an area of surrounding normal bone should be visualised. It is sometimes impractical to achieve this on a periapical film in which case an occlusal or an extra-oral projection may be required.

The radiograph should be carefully examined in a systematic manner. Reference should be made to adjacent anatomical structures, the condition of the surrounding bone and associated periodontal ligament space. The anatomy of the pulp chamber and root canals should be examined, details regarding the presence of caries, features of the coronal restoration, number and anatomy of the roots being particularly important. It must be remembered that a radiograph is only a two dimensional representation of a three-dimensional object and although roots may appear to have mesial or distal curves, they are also likely to curve in buccal or lingual directions. Magnification aids will assist interpretation of the radiograph.

Working length estimation – 'diagnostic' radiographs

These allow the clinician to determine the working length of the tooth, that is, the distance between a fixed coronal reference point and the apical limit of instrumentation. This must be determined for every canal in the tooth to be treated. A combination of knowledge of the expected working length and tactile sensation will assist in initial placement of the diagnostic instrument.

When multiple canals in a single tooth or a multi-rooted tooth are being considered, more than one periapical radiograph may be necessary. In some instances it is possible to take a single radiograph with instruments in different canals. If it is suspected that there are two canals in the same buccolingual plane, these may be distinguished by exposing the film with a mesial and/or a distal angulation on the X-ray tube.

With experience, measurements may be taken from radiographic images although allowances must be made for the inherent linear distortion and magnification present in all radiography. If the apex of the tooth and/or the end of the instrument is not visible then the radiograph is of no diagnostic value.

During diagnostic radiography for working length estimation, it is customary to remove the rubber dam frame to facilitate film placement. The rubber dam and clamp should remain in place during radiography.

Master cone radiographs

Although every care is taken during calculation of the working length, errors can, and do, occur. As a final check before root filling/ obturation, a dry run, or 'cone-fit', radiograph may be taken. A gutta-percha cone is positioned at the full working length and a radiograph taken to ensure that it is in the anticipated place. This radiograph also allows the shape of the preparation to be assessed. Any errors in the preparation or position of the gutta-percha can be corrected before final obturation. Some clinicians also advocate a radiograph part way through obturation, called a 'mid-fill' radiograph, the rationale being that the first cone of gutta-percha may move in the initial stages of obturation.

Follow-up radiographs

Radiographic follow-up is an adjunct to, but should not replace, clinical follow-up. A periapical radiograph is an important aid for evaluating the success or failure of endodontic treatment. The first follow-up radiograph is taken directly after completion of endodontic treatment, preferably by the paralleling technique. Subsequent, follow-up radiographs should be exposed under the same conditions and using the same technique in order to permit comparisons.

The recommended intervals for radiographic follow-up of symptom-free teeth are 6, 12 and 24 months[4]. If resolution is questionable at 2 years, further annual radiographs may be justified. However, it must be remembered that patient exposure to radiation must always be kept as low as reasonably achievable (ALARA).

In cases of teeth that become symptomatic during follow-up, other radiographs may be required according to clinical judgement.

ACCESS CAVITIES

An access cavity is a preparation (usually into the clinical crown) through which treatment of the dental pulp or pulp space is effected. It is essential that the operator has a good understanding of normal tooth and root canal anatomy (Figs 3.1, 3.2).

Objectives

The objectives of preparation of an access cavity are:

- To remove the entire roof of the pulp chamber so that the chamber can be fully debrided and its floor examined to locate canals.
- To facilitate root canal shaping by providing straight-line access to the apical third of the root canals.

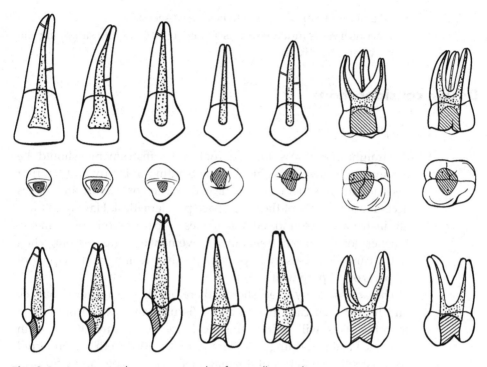

Fig. 3.1 Anatomy and access cavity outline for maxillary teeth.

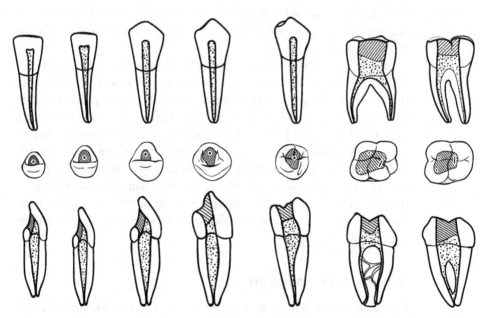

Fig. 3.2 Anatomy and access cavity outline for mandibular teeth.

- To enable a temporary seal to be placed securely.
- To conserve as much tooth tissue as possible (while satisfying the previous objectives).

Design considerations

Preparation form

A straight-line access for the root canal instruments should be achieved whenever possible. Undue bending of instruments during insertion renders them more liable to distortion or fracture and makes access to some part of the pulp space problematic. Having to force an instrument around curves makes a perforation more likely. Furthermore, sufficient freedom of movement of an instrument, when in the canal, is necessary to permit effective cleaning and shaping of all parts of the pulp walls.

The access cavity itself should therefore have a rounded outline and be symmetrically placed about fissures and away from crown margins. This will reduce the incidence of fracture of porcelain crowns. Palatal and lingual openings on anterior teeth are preferred for aesthetic reasons but lingual inclination, especially of lower anteriors (and sometimes premolars), may indicate access cavity preparations involving the labial or buccal surface (Fig. 3.3). Preparation is related to the form and position of the pulp chamber and the root canals extending from it rather than to the overlying fissure pattern.

Unnecessary tissue removal should be avoided because of the functional need to preserve the strength and integrity of root and crown structure. An access cavity through the roof of the pulp chamber significantly weakens the tooth – in the extreme case of a molar with a mesio-occluso-distal preparation, tooth tissue is left only in the furcation area leading to a high risk of fracture if remaining cusps are still in high functional load. Occlusal reduction of a molar undergoing endodontic treatment may be helpful. Subsequent placement of a cuspal coverage restoration will permit restoration of occlusal function. Therefore, the access cavity should be of sufficient size only to satisfy endodontic objectives.

Removal of infected dentine

It is necessary to eliminate any direct source of canal contamination and potential pathway of contamination from the mouth. All unsound restorations and tooth structure should be removed and cavities on the axial wall of the crown thoroughly excavated and, if below the rubber dam, sealed before isolation. If the pulp chamber is opened at this stage it is helpful to protect the floor and the opening(s) to the root canal(s) with a gutta-percha or cotton pellet, which fills the pulp chamber, before placing sealants or new restorations. Total removal of extensive restorations may, however, be undesirable as this could compromise support from weakened residual coronal tissues and make isolation more difficult.

Technique

This may be divided into stages:

- Initial access cavity outline and isolation
- Pulp chamber entry
- Pulp chamber roof removal
- Preparation margin modification
- Cavity refinement
- Irrigation
- Canal orifice opening

Initial access cavity outline and isolation

The initial access stage may be executed before placement of rubber dam (required for isolation) in order to aid orientation.

Pulp chamber entry

Careful reference to preoperative radiographs will give an indication of pulp size or position. Long shank bur designs improve visibility but it is essential that landmarks on the floor of the pulp chamber are maintained. The dust of enamel, dentine or dressing created at this stage may be gently cleared using a three-in-one syringe and aspirator across the mouth of the cavity. Air (or fluids) under pressure should not be blown into the pulp chamber because impaction of debris into the canal may cause blockage and there is a risk of air embolus.

Pulp chamber roof removal

The cavity is then opened up to afford smooth-walled access to the pulp cornua. Extension of the preparation cervicolingually, especially

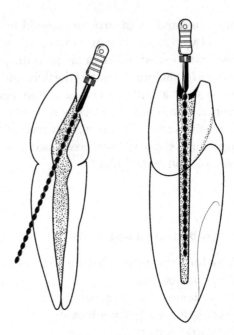

Fig. 3.3 Axial access for a lower incisor. (Straight line access to the root canal requires extension of the access to the incisal edge.)

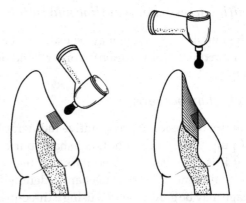

Fig. 3.4 Coronal opening.

in lower incisors, improves access to the buccolingual extremities of an elliptical pulp space (Figs 3.3, 3.4). The use of magnification in the form of loupes or an endodontic microscope has very much enhanced the ease of identification of root canals. Another aid is the use of ultrasonically powered instruments used at low power and without water cooling. Careful use of specially designed tips facilitates the widening of the opening of root canals that may be partially obliterated by calcific material.

Preparation margin modification

Refinement of the preparation margins is carried out, if necessary, to facilitate reproducible positioning of instrument handles against a reliable reference point. Location of the pulp chamber may prove to be difficult under prosthetic crowns. Alignment of the root relative to the crown may be confirmed by imaging techniques, by palpation and by subgingival probing.

Cavity refinement

Creation of pulpally converging walls on opposing aspects of the access cavity is achieved by the use of a safe-ended, non-cutting bur (e.g. a Batt bur) which will prevent damage to the floor of the pulp chamber.

Irrigation

Copious irrigation with sodium hypochlorite (NaOCl) will arrest any haemorrhage, assist in the removal of pulpal remnants (dissolves organic material) and debris obstructions, and assist in the prevention of extension of contamination from crown to root apex (i.e. acts as a disinfectant). A variety of concentrations of sodium hypochlorite (from 0.5% to 5%) are advocated. Higher concentrations act more quickly, although the risk of tissue irritation, if the irrigant is extruded past the apex and into the peri-radicular tissues, is greater. Lower concentrations are also antibacterial, and are less irritant to tissues, but require longer contact times and greater volumes.

Canal orifice opening

The entrances to the canals can be identified with the aid of a sharp probe such as a DG16. There is no sharp delineation between the access preparation stage and canal cleaning and shaping, and to a large extent, the transition stage occurs when initial widening of the canal orifices is carried out. This stage is a natural extension of access preparation, and leads to canal cleaning and shaping. Not withstanding the above, this stage involves use of either hand or

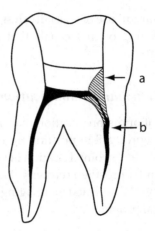

Fig. 3.5 Coronal shaping – ledge removal at (a) gives straight line access to (b).

rotary instruments to widen the orifices of the canals. A sequential series of instruments should be used in decreasing order (larger to smaller), sometimes referred to as 'stepping down'.

The aims of this procedure are to remove any features of the canal wall anatomy which may preclude straight-line access to the canal terminus, to create a greater space in which irrigating solutions are effective and to assist the ease of canal location (Figs 3.4, 3.5). Gates Glidden drills are effective for this procedure (see section on cleaning and shaping).

ENDODONTIC INSTRUMENTS

ISO standardisation

Before a standardised configuration was adopted, endodontic instruments varied greatly from one manufacturer to another. The configuration adopted is that set by the International Organization for Standardization (ISO) and is laid down in ISO specification No. 3630. All ISO hand instruments, along with paper points, silver points and standardised gutta-percha points, conform to this system. ISO standardised files have a cutting length of 16 mm, have a specified diameter at the tip (termed D_1) and increase in diameter by 0.02 mm for each millimetre along the file, so that at the end of the cutting part (16 mm along the file) the diameter (termed D_2) is 0.32 mm greater than at D_1. This is called an .02 taper. Files may vary in length, any extra length is provided by a 'blank' portion. The nominal size of the instrument is based on the diameter of its tip (the diameter at D_1) expressed in hundredths of a millimetre. Thus an ISO size 50 file will have a tip diameter of 0.50 mm.

ISO standardisation also uses a colour for each size, as shown below:

Colour	Nominal Size		
Pink	06		
Grey	08		
Purple	10		
White	15	45	90
Yellow	20	50	100
Red	25	55	110
Blue	30	60	120
Green	35	70	130
Black	40	80	140

Specialised half sizes are colour-coded in the following way:

Purple/Gold	12	White/Gold	17
Yellow/Gold	22	Red/Gold	27
Blue/Gold	32	Green/Gold	37

The length of the instrument is measured in millimetres and is indicated on the packaging. The normal lengths available are 21, 25, 28 and 31 mm.

Endodontic instruments vary according to metal alloy, tip design, mode of manufacture and shape of cutting flutes. There are also a large number of files available that are non-ISO and these vary in taper and length of cutting blade.

Alloys

The properties of root canal instruments are related to the alloy, taper and cross-sectional configuration. Most instruments are constructed either from stainless steel or nickel titanium.

Nickel titanium is composed of approximately 55% nickel and 45% titanium by weight, and instruments constructed from this material are about three times as flexible as stainless steel instruments of the same dimensions. This flexibility facilitates the shaping of very curved canals. Nickel titanium has shape memory; that is, when deformed, it will return to its original shape. This is in contrast to many other metal alloys (for example stainless steel) that, if bent or twisted, may remain permanently deformed. This difference in mechanical properties influences the method of construction. Files made from stainless steel may be made by taking a blank of material, with a rectangular or square cross-section, and twisting it to form cutting flutes. This is not possible with nickel titanium due to its shape memory, so in order to create cutting flutes, the shape must be machined from a blank rather than being twisted.

A major advantage of nickel titanium files is that they are flexible at greater tapers than stainless steel and they may therefore be used in rotary handpieces. A disadvantage is that they are prone to fracture and removal of separated fragments may be difficult.

Hand instruments

Traditionally, hand files were manufactured by twisting square or triangular shafts of metal around their long axis. Recently, computer-assisted machining has enabled the modification of existing file geometries. The principal endodontic instruments are files.

Reamers

Reamers are made from stainless steel and are of square (smaller sizes) or triangular (larger sizes) cross-section. The blank is twisted to create an instrument with cutting flutes at predetermined intervals. These instruments have the disadvantage in that they are relatively inflexible and therefore are restricted to the shaping of canals of round cross-section.

Files

A wide variety of hand files are available, these differ in their configuration and mode of action. Below is a summary of the features of the more common types of files.

Hedström files (Fig. 3.6)

- These are machined from a round tapered blank. A spiral groove is cut into the shank to produce a sharp blade. They are less flexible than K-type instruments and only the smaller sizes may be pre-curved owing to the risk of deformation or fracture.
- Cutting occurs during withdrawal of the file from the canal.
- Hedström files are very efficient in a planing action for removal of dentine.

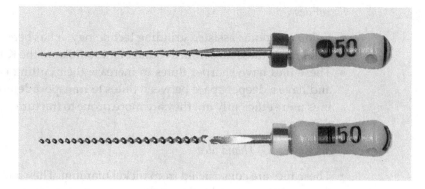

Fig. 3.6 Typical files used in endodontics, Hedström (top) and K-file (bottom).

- They should be inserted slowly with avoidance of rotation (except for a slight rocking motion to aid negotiation).
- They should not be rotated anticlockwise.
- The files are used by withdrawal up each aspect of the root canal in a circumferential filing motion.

K-type files (Fig. 3.6)

- These are probably the most widely used of the 'classical' designs of root canal instrument.
- K-type files are formed by twisting a tapered steel wire of square or triangular cross-section. This method of manufacture results in work hardening and therefore produces a 'springy' instrument with enhanced stiffness for insertion into narrow canals but it will then elastically recoil against the canal wall. These instruments are normally used with a filing action.
- K-type files are less aggressive in planing than the Hedström design.

K-Flex files

- Their cross-sectional geometry is rhomboid to produce alternate high and low flutes so the action is to cut and clean. The high flutes cut and the low flutes allow space for dentinal shavings and more efficient debris removal.
- This cross-sectional configuration results in a reduction in metal, producing increased flexibility without a significant reduction in strength.

FlexoFiles

- Using computer-assisted grinding technology, it has been possible to fabricate these files from a round blank, similar to the K-type file.
- These files have sharper flutes to increase their cutting efficiency and have a deeper space between flutes to transport dentine shavings more efficiently but they are more prone to fracture.

Greater taper (GT) hand files

- These files are constructed from nickel titanium. They are non-ISO files and are available in four sizes with varying taper, increasing from 0.06, 0.08, 0.10 to 0.12; all have a size 20 tip (i.e. 0.20 mm). Gutta-percha cones are available in the same range of tapers, though the terminology used is often (confusingly) different: 0.06 taper is termed fine, 0.08 is fine-medium, 0.10 is medium and 0.12 is medium large.
- GT files are designed to be active in a counter-clockwise direction.
- The most apical extent of a GT file should never engage dentine, rather it should passively follow the canal direction.

Rotary instruments

Gates Glidden drills

The six instruments in this series are made from stainless steel. Each instrument has a long shaft and a flame-shaped cutting head. Gates Glidden drills are ideally used to cut dentine on the withdrawal stroke. They are confined to the straight section of the canal and are used serially and passively in a step-back manner, such that each successively larger drill is worked shorter than the preceding smaller one. They may also be used in a step-down manner. Used properly, these drills are inexpensive, safe and beneficial. However, they must be used with care as they may separate and over-aggressive use may result in perforation of the canal wall.

Nickel titanium rotary instruments

The use of nickel titanium instruments reduces the risk of procedural errors during cleaning and shaping, such as blocks, ledges, transportations and perforations (see later). However, their use is associated with an increased incidence of instrument separation.

There is a wide range of instruments which vary in cross-sectional configuration to some degree. Most have a radial land, that is, a flat planing surface (in contrast to the sharp planing/cutting flutes of twisted hand files), which centralises the instrument in the canal and prevents the instrument from cutting into the canal walls. Cutting of dentine is achieved by engagement of the flutes in the canal walls, debris being theoretically extruded in a coronal direction. Recommendations regarding techniques vary according to the system, but the basic principles remain the same in that the canal should be rendered free from infected material and shaped in such a way that it may be adequately obturated. As is the principle for hand shaping procedures, coronal opening should precede apical and mid-root shaping.

Electronic apex locators

The latest generation of these devices is useful in determining the position of the apical constriction. Many recent models measure impedance rather than electrical resistance, and are less sensitive to ionic solutions within the canal. They should therefore function in the presence of NaOCl, EDTA solution, blood or pus.

Following coronal flaring, one lead from the device is attached to an earthing clip and is positioned on the patient's lip to complete an electrical circuit. The floor of the access cavity and 2–3 mm into the canal is dried. The other lead is clipped to the top of a file. The machine is switched on and the file is slowly advanced into the canal. Some devices show a digital display as the apex is reached and emit an audible bleep. Other devices have a visual display indicating the position at which the end point is reached. The figures should not be taken as an accurate indicator of file tip distance from the apex until zero is reached. If the apex locator is used through a metallic restoration (such as amalgam or a crown), care must be taken to prevent contact of the file with the restoration otherwise shorting of the reading will occur.

When a zero reading is displayed, the distance stop on the file is moved to contact a suitable reference point and the file then removed. The distance between the file tip and the stop is measured and recorded together with the reference point. A diagnostic radiograph is then exposed as described previously.

CLEANING AND SHAPING

Objectives of cleaning and shaping

The objectives of cleaning and shaping are to:

- Create a continuously tapering preparation.
- Maintain the original anatomy.
- Retain the position of the apical foramen.
- Keep the foramen as small as possible.

Step-down is now regarded as the preferred preparation technique[5]. In this method, the coronal part of the canal is prepared before the apical region. The canal working length is determined following the step-down stage and before apical preparation is commenced.

The outcome of this approach to treatment is improved for the following reasons:

- There is better tactile control of instruments in the apical third.
- Pre-enlarged canals can hold a greater volume of irrigant to enhance cleaning.
- Pre-enlarged canals promote the removal of dentine mud.
- Post-treatment problems are reduced as the bulk of bacteria and their toxins will have been removed.
- Identification of the foramen is facilitated.

It is useful to remember that most teeth range from 19 to 25 mm in length. Most crowns are about 10 mm, and most roots range from 9 to 15 mm. The root may be divided into thirds: coronal, middle and apical.

Summary of cleaning and shaping procedures

- Preoperative radiograph
- Administration of a local anaesthetic
- *Rubber dam placement*
- *Access cavity*
- Identification and widening of canal orifices
- Investigation of canal patency
- Coronal two-thirds shaping
- Working length determination (using radiographs and/or an apex locator)
- Apical shaping
- Mid-third shaping and canal refinement

*It may be appropriate to carry out access cavity preparation before isolation.

Negotiation of the coronal two-thirds

Coronal shaping is usefully preceded by negotiation of the canal with small flexible hand files. The aims are to:

- Reveal information about the cross-sectional diameter of a canal and the presence of any constrictions/pulp stones, etc.
- Confirm the presence of straight line access.
- Provide information about the anatomy of the root canal system.

Coronal two-thirds shaping

Coronal flaring (Fig. 3.5) may be accomplished in either a step-back or a crown-down approach. The step-back technique is the sequential use of instruments starting with the smaller sizes and progressing towards the larger. A crown-down approach is the serial use of instruments, starting with the larger and progressing to the smaller. Usually, nickel titanium rotary instruments are used in a crown-down technique, whereas ISO hand files and Gates Glidden drills are best used in a step-back technique for the following reasons:

- Smaller instruments can be placed at a deeper level and cut on the up stroke (thus facilitating the removal of debris).
- The coronal two-thirds can be moved and relocated from the region of the furcation and towards the greatest bulk of dentine.

Working length determination

The working length establishes the apical extent of canal shaping and the end of the root canal filling and should be determined accurately before preparation of the apical third of the canal. When the coronal two-thirds has been pre-enlarged, there is excellent access for negotiation and preparation of the apical one-third.

A file of no smaller than a size 20 should be used as a diagnostic instrument as it may be difficult to distinguish the position of the tip of smaller size files by radiographic means. The file (pre-curved if necessary) is placed in the canal until it has reached this estimated length and a radiograph taken or an apex locator used. A locating stop on the handle of the file should be carefully positioned against a

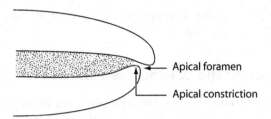

Fig. 3.7 Apical anatomy for working length determination.

reproducible reference point on the tooth to define the coronal aspect of the diagnostic length.

Following working length determination, apical preparation continues by the successive use of progressively larger instruments at the full working length. Copious irrigation and frequent recapitulation with a fine file will prevent build-up of canal debris.

Apical preparation

The terminal extent of shaping should be at the junction between the pulpal and periodontal tissues. This occurs at the apical foramen. Usually, the apical foramen is the narrowest part of the root canal and this narrowing is termed the apical constriction (Fig. 3.7). It has been shown by Kuttler[6] that this position is 0.5–1 mm from the radiographic apex in the majority of cases. However, this is not always the case, for example when the deposition of secondary cementum has occurred. In addition, canal anatomy is variable and the constriction may be at some distance from the foramen. It must also be remembered that the primary root canal does not necessarily exit at the radiographic apex.

Careful apical preparation is fundamental to the success of treatment and several factors should be considered including the apical extent of preparation, relative to the radiographic apex, and the three-dimensional shape and size of the pulp chamber.

Most canals have some degree of curvature. An instrument placed in a curved canal will tend to cut the outer dentine wall to produce a widened, apically directed funnel which is tear-shaped in cross-section. The apical flare is called a zip and the section more coronal to it is called the elbow (Fig. 3.8). To overcome these problems, it is essential that shaping should reflect the canal size and curvature.

The degree to which the apical end of the canal should be prepared is subject to discussion. There is an argument that any significant

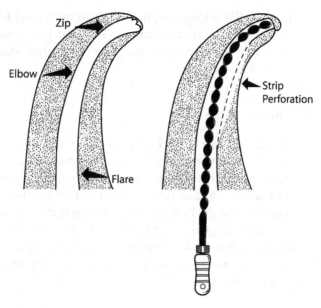

Fig. 3.8 Apical errors.

widening is unnecessary if there has been adequate coronal flaring and adequate irrigation. There is also the risk of zipping or stripping the canal walls when larger size files are used, especially in curved canals. A counter argument is that there needs to be a minimum degree of preparation of the apical third so that infected dentine is removed. It is also easier to fill canals that have a larger apical preparation.

The shape of the apical preparation has also been considered and the terms 'apical seat' (or 'apical box') and 'apical taper' have been described. The fundamental philosophy is that if the terminal end of the canal is wide, then creation of an apical seat reduces the risk of overextension of the filling material. However, if the canal is fine and curved in its apical extremity, then production of an apical seat runs the risk of creation of apical stripping or zip formation.

Whichever method is adopted, it should be possible to place a spreader (a tapered, blank, pointed instrument used to push gutta-percha to one side when obturating) to within 2 mm of the radio-graphic apex.

'Stepping back' by using sequentially increasing size files at 1-mm increments short of the working length produces an apical taper. In between each larger file, the master apical file (or a fine file) is inserted to the full working length and irrigation is used to eliminate debris; this is termed 'recapitulation'. The step back process is continued until this portion of the preparation reaches and blends with the coronal preparation.

Patency filing

Despite the careful and frequent use of irrigation, there is a risk that the accumulation of canal debris may result in apical blockage. It has been argued that this may be avoided by penetration of the apical constriction of the canal with a small file during the shaping procedure[7,8]. This is thought both to direct the irrigating solution apically and also to dislodge the apical debris into the canal. Subsequent irrigation results in its removal. A counter argument is that this only applies to the main canal and there is a risk of inoculating infected canal contents further apically.

Mid-third shaping

The ideal shape for obturation purposes is that of a continuously tapering cone[9]. However, over-shaping brings with it the risk of weakening the tooth structure or stripping the canal walls. On the other hand, under-shaping may result in the accumulation of residual infected dentine and debris.

Curved canals – the balanced force technique

There are a number of techniques for avoiding problems associated with curved canals including step-back, pre-curving of files and anticurvature filing[10] (the preferential filing of the outer curve of the canal to reduce the chance of a strip perforation). The Balanced Force Technique[11] is the use of instruments in a step-down manner to initiate pre-enlargement procedures and to gain access to the apical third efficiently. This is basically a reaming technique and adopts a 60–90° clockwise action, for file insertion and dentine engagement, followed by a 120–180° anticlockwise movement with apically directed pressure for dentine removal. A final clockwise movement allows the file flutes to be filled with debris and removed from the canal. This method is said to be efficient and less likely to cause stripping of the canal walls due to the instrument being centrally located. There is also thought to be less risk of apical extrusion of debris.

Smear layer management

When the blades of any file engage and cut dentine, a smear layer of organic and inorganic debris forms on the walls of the preparation. Whether or not to remove the smear layer or leave it intact is still debated. If the smear layer is removed then a tighter interface between the obturation materials and the dentine walls is possible. If the smear layer is left, then the root canal system is incompletely sealed and the potential for microleakage increases. EDTA in its aqueous form, flooded into well-shaped preparations has been shown to remove the inorganic component of the smear layer, and when used in conjunction with sodium hypochlorite will eliminate the smear layer.

INTER-APPOINTMENT MEDICAMENTS

In asymptomatic teeth in which complications are not anticipated, cleaning, shaping and filling can be carried out in one visit. However, as it has been shown that elimination of intra-canal infection cannot be achieved at one treatment session, the use of intra-canal medicaments and filling of the canals at a second visit is justified[12].

Theoretically, therefore, teeth with apical periodontitis should have a better prognosis when treated in more than one visit and when an intra-canal medicament is placed. However, this hypothesis is not always supported clinically as some studies indicate that teeth with apical periodontitis can perform well when treated in one visit[12,13].

The requirements of an inter-appointment medicament are that it should be:

- Intact for the period of dressing
- Easy to apply and remove
- Antibacterial
- Eliminate any space for bacterial growth

In order to place an inter-appointment medicament, the canal is rendered clean and dry following cleaning and shaping before being filled with the paste material. This may be delivered on a pre-measured paper point, file or Lentulo spiral filler to the anatomic apex. Careful application of pressure using a cotton pellet ensures that the paste is condensed towards the apex. Excess material is blotted dry from the pulp chamber and the cavity sealed with a temporary cement overlaid with a more rigid material.

A variety of materials have been proposed for this purpose including antiseptic pastes and other relatively toxic solutions and tinctures.

Calcium hydroxide

Calcium hydroxide has many of the properties of an ideal medicament. A non-setting paste of calcium hydroxide may either be made by mixing a powder form and sterile water, or purchased as a commercial product. It has the following properties:

- Strongly alkaline
- Antimicrobial and antibacterial
- Has low solubility
- Controls seepage of inflammatory exudates
- Induces calcific barrier formation

Iodine compounds

Most organisms are susceptible to calcium hydroxide, but this material is not always effective in teeth of complex root morphology in which complete filling of lateral canals cannot be guaranteed. In addition, some organisms, and particularly those implicated in re-treatment cases, such as *Enterococcus faecalis*, are resistant to calcium hydroxide. They are, however, susceptible to iodine-containing compounds such as iodine potassium iodide. The presence of a smear layer inhibits penetration, hence the rationale for removal of the smear layer before placement of the inter-appointment medicament. Iodine-containing compounds have good penetration effects, and will diffuse into dentinal tubules and lateral canals, but they are also short-lasting. It is therefore considered that a mixture of calcium hydroxide and 5% iodine potassium iodide is an appropriate inter-appointment medicament in re-treatment cases.

Steroid–antibiotic compounds

Commercial combinations of a steroid with an antibiotic are available and are used by some practitioners to alleviate the symptoms of an acute or terminal pulpitis. The steroid component suppresses the inflammatory response while the antibiotic addresses the microbial infection. However, such products should not be used as an alternative to meticulous cleaning and shaping procedures.

Mineral trioxide aggregate

Although not an inter-appointment medicament, mineral trioxide aggregate (MTA) is an innovative material that appears to induce the formation of new bone and is used for perforation repair. Root perforations are an unfortunate recognised hazard associated with endodontic treatment and post-space preparation. The communication is likely to stimulate an inflammatory response and consequent resorption in the adjacent bone. It is therefore important to seal the defect as soon as possible. This is achieved by placement of a pellet of MTA cement over the defective site and by dressing the tooth. At a second visit, the temporary material is removed and the MTA is checked to ensure that it has set. The canals may then be obturated conventionally and the tooth kept under clinical and radiographic review.

OBTURATION (ROOT FILLING)

Rationale

The pulp space of a non-vital tooth is a potential reservoir for the stagnation and degeneration of tissue fluids to occur, and may act as a source of initiation and maintenance of periapical disease. If these stagnant and necrotic substances are contaminated with micro-organisms there is a potentially inaccessible source of persistent and progressive disease. To prevent this from happening, complete, three-dimensional obturation of the cleaned and shaped root canal with an impervious filling should be carried out to seal off communication between the pulp space and periodontal membrane.

Objectives

The objectives of filling, or 'obturating', the canal space are:

- To prevent percolation of peri-radicular exudates into the pulp space via the apical foramina or lateral canals.
- To prevent proliferation and spread of micro-organisms from the canal into the surrounding tissues.
- To seal the canal from coronal leakage.
- To encompass any residual bacteria.

Sealers

Gutta-percha is the most commonly used root canal filling material but does not adhere to dentine. Warm gutta-percha may contract away from the root canal walls, leaving a potential space into which fluids may percolate. There is therefore a need to use a sealant material that bridges the gap between the filling and the walls of the canal and fills any potential spaces into which micro-organisms may proliferate.

A sealer may fulfil any one or more of the following functions:

- Acts as a luting agent
- Fills any discrepancy between the canal walls and core material
- Fills any discrepancy between gutta-percha points
- Acts as a lubricant
- Acts as a bactericidal agent
- Fills any lateral canals

Requirements

A sealer should have the following properties:

- Be capable of achieving a thin film
- Have high tissue tolerance
- Be of uniform consistency
- Have good rheological properties
- Be of low solubility
- Have an adequate working time

Groups

There is a variety of sealers available, and these may be simply split according to their constituents:

- Zinc oxide based
- Calcium hydroxide based
- Resin sealers
- Glass-ionomer sealers

In the initial setting phase, sealers may be cytotoxic; hence, overextension of the sealer beyond the confines of the canal should be avoided.

Gutta-percha

Gutta-percha has been used for more than 100 years. It is a form of rubber mixed with zinc oxide and other agents. Although not ideal, its advantages are that it is inert, is dimensionally stable, is non-allergenic, antibacterial, non-staining, radiopaque, compactable, may be softened by heat and organic solvents and may be removed from the canal.

Filling techniques

There are various techniques. These may be divided into:

* Solid gutta-percha techniques
* Softened gutta-percha techniques

Gutta-percha may be softened using either heat or solvents

Solid core techniques

Solid core techniques may utilise a single cone of gutta-percha or may employ lateral condensation of multiple cones of gutta-percha. For these methods, a gutta-percha cone is selected to match the size of the apical preparation, i.e. a master cone of the same size as the master apical file is chosen. Although a master cone is selected to match the size of the master apical file, the apical preparation may be larger than the nominal size due to the filing action of the file. Therefore, the selected master cone may, in fact, be a loose fit. In order to achieve a good friction fit (termed 'tug-back'), the tapered master cone is shortened slightly so that it has a slightly larger diameter at its end. Several trial fits may be necessary to obtain the required tug-back at the correct length.

In the single cone method, the gutta-percha cone is selected to match the canal preparation dimension. Although this is a quick technique, the main disadvantage is that only canals of circular dimension may be adequately filled and this rarely represents the true clinical situation. Should this method be used in non-circular canals, there will not be a three-dimensional fill.

In the lateral condensation technique (the favoured method for solid core techniques), a master gutta-percha cone, corresponding to the apical preparation dimension, is placed in position, alongside which are condensed additional accessory gutta-percha points. The advantage is that the canal may be filled in all dimensions, the final material being a mass of gutta-percha points joined by a thin layer of sealant material. This is, however, a technique-sensitive method, it can be time consuming and is not appropriate in cases of internal resorption, for example. It must also be remembered that filling of lateral canals by sealant cannot be guaranteed.

A gutta-percha point of the same size as the master apical file should wedge slightly at 0.5–1.0 mm short of the full working length and a 'dry run' root filling radiograph is useful to confirm its position. Measurement of a spreader (a tapered, blank, pointed instrument used to push the gutta-percha to one side) to 2 mm short of the working length ensures that apically directed pressure will not result in overextension of the gutta-percha.

The walls of the canal to 2 mm short of the apex should be coated with an even, thin film of sealant and this also facilitates placement of the master gutta-percha point by acting as a lubricant. Controlled placement of the coated master cone allows extrusion of excess sealer in a coronal direction before it is seated with firm pressure and a twisting action. Insertion of either a hand or finger spreader to the depth indicated by the stop, alongside the master cone, pushing it to one side and oscillating and withdrawing the spreader results in creation of space for the placement of additional wedging or lateral cones. When excess filling material at the base of the pulp chamber has been seared off using a hot 'plastic' instrument to the level of the canal orifice, a check root filling radiograph should be carefully assessed to confirm that the root has been adequately obturated.

Softened gutta-percha methods

Several methods have been described to plasticise gutta-percha. These may be divided into:

- Heat applied inside the canal
  - — warm vertical condensation
  - — warm lateral condensation
  - — thermomechanical compaction
- Heat applied outside the canal
  - — injection technique
- Carrier-based methods
  - — heat applied outside the canal
  - — mechanical sources of heat
- Solvent methods

Warm lateral condensation involves the use of a heated spreader applied to a master gutta-percha cone inside the canal. Heat may be derived either from an external source (such as a warm Bunsen) or from a thermostatically heated spreader. Pressure is applied and the heated mass is adapted to the canal walls. The warm spreader is removed and a cold spreader creates space for further cones to be added. This process is repeated.

Warm vertical condensation involves a process similar to the above, except vertically directed forces are applied. The disadvantage is that there is a danger of overextension of filling material and sealant if there is not good resistance to apical extrusion.

Gutta-percha may be warmed in a thermostatically heated delivery gun and applied/injected into the canal via a needle[14]. A cold vertical condenser is used to compact the material. This method is particularly useful to fill root canal systems of non-conventional morphology (e.g. internal resorption). Again, there is a danger of overextension of material in the absence of a positive apical stop. Prior placement of a master cone precludes this potential problem.

Use of a mechanically operated thermomechanical compacter softens a gutta-percha cone which is adapted to the canal walls. Placement of a gutta-percha cone is essential to preclude overextension of material. Disadvantages include the risk of instrument separation, results may be inconsistent and even if a master cone is placed, apical extrusion of material may result.

Coronal seal

Studies have shown that the quality of the coronal seal has a significant effect on the outcome of endodontic treatment with coronal leakage being associated with a less favourable result[15,16]. A number of studies have shown that coronal leakage is reduced if the smear layer is removed[17]. Leakage will also be prevented if an adhesive restoration is placed in the coronal aspect of the tooth, hence the justification for placement of a resin-modified glass-ionomer material over the gutta-percha followed by provision of a well-sealed temporary or permanent filling.

REFERENCES

1. Kakehashi S., Stanley H.R. and Fitzgerald R.J. The effects of surgical exposures of dental pulps in germ-free and conventional laboratory rats. *Oral Surg Oral Med Oral Pathol*, 1965; **20**: 340–9.
2. Faculty of General Dental Practitioners [FGDP]. Radiographs in endodontics. In: *Selection Criteria for Dental Radiography*, 2nd edn. London, FGDP(UK), 2004, pp. 63–71.
3. Fava L.R. and Dummer P.M. Periapical radiographic techniques during endodontic diagnosis and treatment. *Int Endod J*, 1997; **30**: 250–61.

4. Consensus report of the European Society of Endodontology on quality guidelines for endodontic treatment. *Int Endod J*, 1994; **27**: 115–24.

5. Goerig A.C., Michelich R.J. and Schultz H.H. Instrumentation of root canals in molars using the step-down technique. *J Endod*, 1982; **8**: 550–4.

6. Kuttler Y. Microscopic investigation of root apices. *J Am Dent Assoc*, 1955; **50**: 544–52.

7. Schilder H. Cleaning and shaping the root canal. *Dent Clin North Am*, 1974; **18**: 269–96.

8. Buchanan L.S. Working length and apical patency: the control factors. *Endod Rep*, 1987; 16–20.

9. West J.D. and Roane J.B. Cleaning and shaping the root canal system. In: Cohen, S. and Burns, R.C. (eds) *Pathways of the Pulp*, 7th edn. London, Mosby, 1988, pp. 203–57.

10. Abou-Rass M., Frank A.L. and Glick D.H. The anticurvature filing method to prepare the curved root canal. *J Am Dent Assoc*, 1980; **101**: 792–4.

11. Roane J.B., Sabala C.L. and Duncanson M.G., Jr. The 'balanced force' concept for instrumentation of curved canals. *J Endod*, 1985; **11**: 203–11.

12. Sjogren U., Figdor D., Persson S. and Sundqvist G. Influence of infection at the time of root filling on the outcome of endodontic treatment of teeth with apical periodontitis. *Int Endod J*, 1997; **30**: 297–306.

13. Pekruhn R.B. The incidence of failure following single-visit endodontic therapy. *J Endod*, 1986; **12**: 68–72.

14. Yee F.S., Marlin J., Krakow A.A. and Gron P. Three-dimensional obturation of the root canal using injection-moulded, thermoplasticized dental gutta-percha. *J Endod*, 1977; **3**: 168–74.

15. Ray H.A. and Trope M. Periapical status of endodontically treated teeth in relation to the technical quality of the root filling and the coronal restoration. *Int Endod J*, 1995; **28**: 12–18.

16. Saunders W.P. and Saunders E.M. Coronal leakage as a cause of failure in root-canal therapy: a review. *Endod Dent Traumatol*, 1994; **10**: 105–8.

17. Taylor J.K., Jeansonne B.G. and Lemon R.R. Coronal leakage: effects of smear layer, obturation technique, and sealer. *J Endod*, 1997; **23**: 508–12.

Endodontics – further considerations

TRAUMA

Injuries to teeth are common. In a prospective study where all dental injuries occurring from birth to the age of 14 were registered, it was found that 30% of children had sustained injuries to the primary dentition and 22% to the permanent dentition[1]. These statistics are age-related. In the primary dentition, the prevalence of injuries ranges from 31 to 40% in boys and from 16 to 30% in girls. In the permanent dentition, the prevalence of dental trauma in boys ranges from 12 to 33% compared with 4 to 19% in girls. Most injuries affect the maxillary incisors and in the majority of cases, only one tooth is affected. An increased overjet with prominent incisors and incompetent lips have been found to be predisposing factors.

Prevention

Patients with an increased maxillary overjet have a significantly greater risk of traumatic dental injuries. An additional trauma factor is insufficient lip protection. Collision sports have been the cause of many injuries to the head and neck. It is clear that protection of the oral and dental tissues is needed for all participants in active contact sports. This is best provided by a gum shield made by a dentist.

Effects

Traumatic injuries may affect the teeth in various ways including:

- Chipped enamel or enamel infraction
- Fracture into dentine

81

- Fracture exposing pulp
- Fracture involving both crown and root
- Root fracture
- Avulsion
- Tooth loosened in socket (intrusion/extrusion/luxated)

History

This should include a medical and dental history, age, time of accident, cause, pain, previous trauma history, loss of consciousness and treatment already carried out for the injury including information about the storage conditions of the tooth.

Pulp sensibility testing

Pulp testing following traumatic injuries can be unreliable. These procedures require cooperation and a relaxed patient in order to avoid false responses. Pulp sensibility testing, however, *is* important at the time of injury for establishing a point of reference for evaluating pulpal status at later follow-up examinations. It is essential to review traumatised teeth clinically and radiographically before instituting endodontic therapy.

Radiographs

These are important for initial diagnosis and later comparisons. Films must be dry, and radiographs should also be available of the contralateral teeth. It is essential to look for root development, fractures, widening of the periodontal membrane space, size of the pulp, proximity of the pulp to any fracture, damage to adjacent teeth, coincidental pathology and foreign bodies.

Treatment options

Chipped enamel

The degree of damage depends on energy dissipation. Infractions usually require no treatment. The trauma may have affected the periapical tissues and there is the possibility that the pulp will become non-vital. Pulp sensibility tests should be performed 3-monthly for 1 year and radiographs 6-monthly for at least three recalls.

Fracture into dentine

As dentine is exposed, there are two priorities – to protect the exposed dentine and prevent possible migration of a tooth that has lost contact with its neighbours. This may be done with a directly bonded restoration or fragment.

Fracture exposing pulp

A complicated crown fracture implies exposure of the pulp to the oral environment. Healing is not spontaneous and untreated exposures lead to total pulp necrosis. The aim of pulp capping or pulpotomy treatment is to preserve a vital pulp, which is biologically walled off by a continuous hard tissue barrier. The maturity of the tooth is most significant. It is agreed that the exposed pulp should be maintained in young teeth with incomplete root formation and removed in mature teeth when constriction of the apical foramen allows adequate obturation of the root canal.

Fracture involving both crown and root

A decision must be taken as to whether the tooth can be root filled and a satisfactory restoration ultimately provided, or the tooth should be extracted.

Root fracture

Although the reported incidence of these injuries is low the true number may well be higher as 'unknown' fractures are sometimes revealed. They most commonly occur in the middle third of a fully erupted, fully formed tooth and healing is possible along similar lines to healing of a fractured bone.

The avulsed tooth

This most commonly occurs in males, in upper incisors and particularly in younger patients with protrusive teeth. In the majority of cases, reimplantation is carried out but no guarantee of success should be given to the patient. Replanted teeth are often subject to resorption which may be either inflammatory or replacement (ankylosis).

The loose tooth

Any tooth loosened in its socket may become non-vital as a result of damage to apical blood vessels. Regular reviews are thus required to assess clinical and radiographic changes.

Splinting

Splints are used to stabilise teeth loosened in their sockets, teeth with root fractures, teeth lost (avulsed) and replanted, fractures of the alveolus and fractures of facial bones. Splinting is ideally provided directly by joining adjacent teeth together with an adhesive restorative material (such as glass-ionomer cement or bonded composite), or a piece of wire (for example orthodontic wire) retained on the teeth by an adhesive restorative material or orthodontic brackets. Other techniques such as the use of interdental/eyelet wires have been described, though these may be traumatic to the gingival tissues and may extrude a tooth if inappropriately applied. Teeth may also be splinted with a removable appliance constructed on a cast. The most suitable method will vary in each case, but generally that which is least intrusive whilst fulfilling its role should be used.

The duration of splinting varies depending on the type of injury. Where soft tissue only has been injured (for example a luxation injury) then the period of splinting may be as little as one week or less. Where there is significant hard tissue injury (for example alveolar fracture or root fracture) a much longer period of wear (up to 3 months) is required. Whatever method of splinting is employed, care must be taken that the splint is neither too rigid nor placed for too long as both these will increase the risk of ankylosis.

Injuries to developing teeth

The close relationship between the apices of primary teeth and their permanent successors explains why injuries are easily transmitted from the primary to the permanent dentition. Traumatic injuries to developing teeth may influence their future growth and maturation. When the injury occurs during the initial stages of development, enamel formation can be seriously disturbed owing to interference with a number of stages in ameloblast development.

Resorption

Transient root resorption occurs frequently in traumatised teeth[2] and in those undergoing orthodontic treatment. It is normally without clinical significance. Pressure resorption in the permanent dentition seen during tooth eruption is also seen in orthodontic movement of teeth[3] and usually manifests as a shortening of the roots. It may be quite destructive if diagnosed late.

Root resorption sustained by infection is the most important clinical condition from an endodontic point of view. It can occur either on the root surface (external resorption), or in the root canal (internal resorption). Replacement or endosteal root resorption is seen in teeth that have suffered dentoalveolar ankylosis because of necrosis of the periodontal ligament.

Internal root resorption

It has been shown that bacterial infection is a prerequisite for internal resorption[4]. This process seems to be elicited by irritation from bacteria or their products within the dental tubules derived from caries, fractures or anatomical defects. Sometimes, resorptive defects are noted radiographically in root-filled teeth and this may be attributed to percolation of oral fluids via a defective coronal restoration or periodontal pocket and lateral canals etc. When seen radiographically, internal resorption is a definite indication that endodontic treatment is required. Clinically, there is necrosis in the pulp chamber and in the root canal to a level coronal to the resorption lacunae. Root treatment is complicated by the problems associated with removal of tissue from a resorptive defect and any remnants may contribute to failure. The treatment of choice is to use sodium hypochlorite as an irrigant and to dress the canal with calcium hydroxide paste, replacing at 2–3-week intervals before filling with gutta-percha. A thermo-softened filling method may be indicated if there is extensive resorption.

Cervical root resorption

This appears to follow injury to the cervical attachment apparatus of the tooth. It is most often an inflammatory type of resorption and if local necrosis of the periodontal ligament takes place ankylosis may ensue. Cervical resorption is not a pulpal reaction, but is of importance if it penetrates the root canal. It then becomes an endodontic problem.

External inflammatory root resorption

This is a commonly occurring complication following trauma to the teeth. The condition can be recognised radiographically as a peri-radicular radiolucent area encompassing areas of the root and adjacent alveolar bone. It is important that endodontic therapy is instituted as soon as there are clinical or radiographic signs that resorption is in progress as the resorptive process may destroy the tooth in a few months. Treatment is similar to that for treatment of non-vital teeth and the success is related to removal of the necrotic pulp. There is clinical evidence that long-term treatment with calcium hydroxide provides the most predictable results[5].

Replacement resorption

Damage to the periodontal structure can result in surface resorption when the root surface is seen to demonstrate the presence of super-ficial lacunae with new cementum formation. It has been proposed that this is a response to localised injury to the periodontal ligament. This may be self-limiting and spontaneously repair. Extension of this process may result in direct union between bone and root substance. Clinically, dentoalveolar ankylosis will be recognised because of the lack of tooth mobility. Radiographically, there will be an absence of periodontal space. Also, there may be a 'moth eaten' appearance of the root. There is at present no treatment for this condition although the speed with which the root is replaced by bone is relatively slow and may take several years.

PERIO-ENDO CONNECTIONS

The pulp and the periodontal ligament are closely connected via:

* The apex or apices
* Other vascular channels (e.g. lateral and furcation canals)
* Dentinal tubules

Therefore, it is not surprising that there should be a relationship between diseases of the pulp and the periodontium. In determining the treatment for a particular tooth it is essential to know whether the initial lesion is of periodontal or endodontic origin (Fig. 4.1).

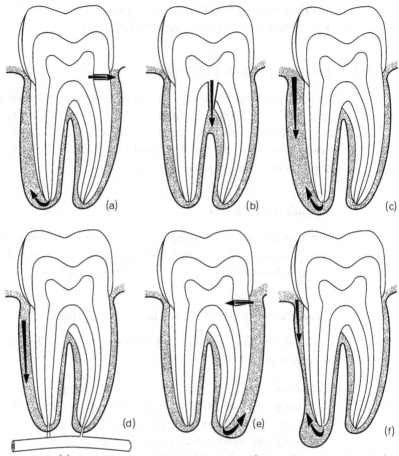

(a) sinus through periodontal membrane (from apex or lateral canal)
(b) from apex or accessory canal with furcation involvement
(c) from apex with concurrent periodontal pocketing
(d) progression of periodontitis to apical involvement with vital pulp
(e) secondary endodontic involvement via lateral canal
(f) true coalescence to form a combined lesion

Fig. 4.1 Origin and passage of infection in combined perio-endo lesions.

Classifications

The following classifications of endodontic and periodontal lesions have been proposed:

- Lesions of endodontic origin
- Periodontal lesions
- Primary endodontic/secondary periodontal

- Primary periodontal/secondary endodontic
- Combined endodontic/periodontal lesions

Lesions of endodontic origin

Lesions of endodontic origin are simple periapical or lateral periodontal granulomas (chronic apical/lateral periodontitis characterised by aggregations of macrophages, lymphocytes and plasma cells) and abscesses (acute apical/lateral periodontitis) recognised by the usual clinical and radiographic features.

Periodontal lesions

Periodontal lesions are diagnosed on the basis of generally accepted criteria including derangement of gingival architecture and loss of gingival attachment as demonstrated by pocket probing and radiographs.

Primary endodontic/secondary periodontal

Endodontic disease may masquerade as periodontal disease in several ways:

- Drainage of a periapical lesion via the periodontal ligament, perhaps perforating the gingivae at, or near to, the mucogingival junction, or exiting via the gingival crevice.
- Endodontic lesions formed via lateral canals at places on the root surface other than at the apex.
- Lateral perforation of the root during root canal or post preparation leading to a lateral periodontal abscess which may drain via the gingival crevice.
- Endodontic lesions in furcation areas formed via 'lateral' canals leading to abscesses, sinuses and radiographic bone loss, which may look like periodontal disease.

Primary periodontal/secondary endodontic

Chronic periodontitis may lead to pulpal disease by means of direct bacterial invasion, or trauma during root surface instrumentation as part of treatment. Chemicals and obtundents used to relieve dentine sensitivity may irritate the pulp, as may the exposure of root surfaces by gingival recession. There is some disagreement in the literature about whether this really happens, mainly because many teeth with significant periodontal disease also have large restorations, so it is impossible to know whether the pulpal lesion was caused by caries, restoration or periodontitis.

Combined endodontic/periodontal lesions

Combined endodontic/periodontal lesions may be:

- Independent of one another
- Coalescing

Differential diagnosis

Differential diagnosis is based upon interpretation of information gained from the following:

- History:
  — pain (duration and character)
- Clinical examination:
  — swelling (site, type and character)
  — discharge (type of fluid, blood, pus etc.)
  — percussion (gentle percussion in several directions)
  — mobility
- Special tests:
  — vitality/sensibility testing (electrical and/or thermal, mechanical)
  — periodontal probing
  — test cavity
  — radiographs (parallax views if necessary)

Treatment planning

In determining the treatment to be provided, an assessment of the vitality of the tooth in question is required. In some instances, it may not be clear whether the pulp is vital or not. In these cases a judgement must be made based on the available evidence from the history and clinical appearance (including special investigations) and treatment instigated. The options for treatment are summarised below:

- Pulp judged to be healthy:
  — periodontal therapy
  — reassessment: if unsuccessful commence endodontic

therapy.
If successful no further treatment.
- Pulp judged to be unhealthy:
  — endodontic therapy
  — reassessment: if unsuccessful commence periodontal therapy. If successful no further treatment.

ELECTIVE ENDODONTICS

Elective devitalisation is the procedure that involves the purposeful extirpation of healthy (i.e. non-inflamed, non-infected) pulpal tissue as a prelude or aid to provision of a restoration. Pulpal tissues comprise part of a dentino-pulpal complex and can normally respond dynamically to stimuli and may play a role in proprioception. As such, the needless removal of this important tissue should be avoided; however there are certain situations in which elective devitalisation may still have a role.

Rationale for devitalisation

In general terms, the basis for elective devitalisation of a tooth may be due to biological considerations, mechanical considerations or as an aid to specific treatments.

Biological considerations

A tooth that has an extensive restoration is likely to have had multiple previous restorations, the placement of each having caused trauma to the pulpal tissues. These injurious insults to the tooth are thought to be cumulative[6] (termed 'stressed pulp syndrome') and further restorations or preparation for an indirect restoration will further stress the pulpal health. In such a situation the likelihood of subsequent loss of vitality is obviously increased. When the tooth in question is to be restored indirectly, the problems of performing root canal treatment through the restoration are axiomatic. The problems are further compounded if the unit in question forms part of a larger restoration, such as a bridge retainer. In addition to the problems of performing root canal treatment, the indirect restoration itself is also compromised with lower survival[7]. Given the situation of an extensively restored tooth that requires restoration with an indirect restoration and has uncertain or doubtful vitality, it is sometimes prudent to perform root canal treatment before provision of the restoration.

There are also a number of other situations in which elective devitalisation may be performed for biological reasons: continued sensitivity not amenable or not responsive to treatment, evidence of progressively sclerosing canals, root resorption and treatment for periodontal disease that involves root amputation or hemisection.

Mechanical considerations

When insufficient coronal dentine remains to provide for retention and resistance, placement of a restoration is problematic. In this situation, placement of a corono-radicular core will allow for the retentive and resistance form to be provided by the radicular dentine. This may be achieved through placement of the restorative material alone (such as an 'amalgam–dowel core') or in combination with an intra-radicular post. Obviously, using the radicular dentine for retention will necessitate root canal treatment.

When a tooth is extensively restored and/or has a poor crown to root ratio due to bone loss arising from periodontal disease, elective devitalisation and crown reduction will reduce the influence of any lateral forces acting upon the tooth. This is of particular relevance when the tooth in question is a potential abutment for a partial denture. The reduced tooth may then be utilised as an overdenture abutment, providing support and stability for the prosthesis as well as maintenance of alveolar bone.

Aid to treatment

Occasional situations may arise in which devitalisation of teeth will aid provision of treatment. Although uncommon, such situations include gross adjustment of occlusal irregularities or major realignment of tooth axes.

Risks and complications

Although the above arguments for elective devitalisation are persuasive for some situations, such a procedure is not without its drawbacks. The primary consideration is that the success of root canal treatment cannot be guaranteed. Despite advances in endodontic treatment, the potential for failure of the root canal treatment should be weighed carefully against the risks/problems of restoring the tooth without devitalising it. Although root canal treatment and placement of an intra-radicular post was once thought to strengthen a root (even being advocated for otherwise healthy teeth that were planned to act as bridge abutments!) it is now accepted that this will, in fact, pre-dispose to root fracture[8]. Although there is no conclusive evidence that endodontically treated teeth are more brittle, the procedure itself will weaken the tooth due to the amount of coronal and radicular dentine that will be removed.

Teeth that have been root filled have shown poor performance as bridge abutments and especially so if an intra-radicular post is present. Such poor performance is even more likely when root-filled teeth support a distal extension, whether this is a removable partial denture or a cantilever bridge[9,10]. This may in part be as a result of a decreased proprioceptive mechanism following pulpectomy.

It should also be remembered that elective devitalisation before definitive treatment will increase the time required to complete the treatment and also increase costs.

Making a decision

Whether or not to perform elective devitalisation should not be an empirical decision but each tooth should be assessed individually. Such assessment should include not only a careful clinical examina-tion regarding current status of the tooth, but also the history of the tooth. Radiographs and sensibility (vitality) testing are essential aids. The aim of assessment is to determine the risks involved in not devi-talising the tooth, primarily with respect to the chance of requiring root canal treatment once the definitive restoration has been placed, compared with the increase in complications such as failure of the root canal treatment and potential for higher failure of the tooth or restoration itself.

In situations in which elective devitalisation is being considered, alternative treatment options should be explored. Such options may include surgical crown lengthening, orthodontic movement or use of a bonded restoration. Advances in multi-purpose bonding systems may allow for placement of restorations (direct or indirect) whereby retention is provided solely by the bond to tooth structure. Although little long-term clinical data exist for this technique it has obvious advantages if the longevity of the tooth can be increased.

There will be situations in which significant doubt exists over the potential for continued vitality of a tooth or when a restoration cannot be placed without utilising radicular dentine to provide retention.

Careful planned elective devitalisation and appropriate restoration may prove wise in such instances.

RESTORATION OF THE ROOT-FILLED TOOTH

Once a tooth has undergone endodontic treatment it is then necessary to restore the tooth in order to:

- Provide a coronal seal (this has a significant effect on the outcome of the endodontic treatment)[11,12].
- Return the tooth to function.
- Protect the remaining tooth from fracture.

In most instances, teeth that have undergone endodontic treatment will be doubly weakened. By the very nature of factors resulting in loss of vitality, the majority of endodontically treated teeth will already have suffered from a significant loss of tooth structure as a result of the cumulative ravages of caries and previous restoration. To enable endodontic access these already weakened teeth then have a significant further amount of tooth structure removed. In addition, it has been suggested that endodontically treated teeth are more brittle. More recent studies dispute this, though some change in physical properties do occur.

Anterior teeth

In anterior teeth, the amount of tooth structure removed to gain access to the pulp space is not overly large and does not have a large effect on the fracture resistance of the tooth. Thus for most anterior teeth, the only restorative need is to provide a coronal seal and return to function. In many cases this may be achieved simply by removing the obturant (gutta-percha) to a level slightly below the gingival margin or cemento-enamel margin, placing a 'sealing' material (such as a resin-modified glass-ionomer cement) 1–2 mm thick and then restoring the access cavity with a resin composite (Fig. 4.2). Where the existing loss of tooth structure is extensive, more attention should be given to the retention of the 'core' restoration and an indirect restoration such as a full coverage crown should be provided.

Posterior teeth

The restoration of root-filled posterior teeth is complicated by the

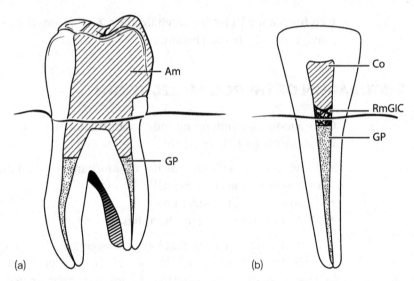

Fig. 4.2 Direct restoration of (a) posterior and (b) anterior root filled teeth (Am = amalgam, GP = gutta-percha, Co = composite, RmGIC = resin-modified glass-ionomer cement).

axial stress placed on any restoration distal to the canines. The preparation of the access cavity and removal of the roof of the pulp chamber acts to increase the stresses at the base of the cusps during function and predisposes these cusps to fracture. In addition, in most root-filled posterior teeth, removal of caries and defective restorations will have resulted in disruption of the marginal ridge, which further weakens the tooth. The overall result of this is that the compromised cuspal tissue cannot withstand the 'wedging' forces developed during function and is liable to fracture[13].

When restoring endodontically treated posterior teeth, consideration needs to be given to the high risk of cuspal fracture. Although some protection may be given to weakened cusps by placing a bonded restoration[14], in any tooth in which the existing restoration and access cavity combined involves more than the occlusal surface, some form of cuspal protection is required. As discussed in Chapter 5, although cuspal coverage may be provided with a direct restoration, practically this need is best served by provision of an indirect restoration that overlays the cusps at risk of fracture. Thus most endodontically treated posterior teeth require restoration with a suitable core followed by provision of an indirect restoration such as a crown or cuspal coverage inlay.

The choice of core restoration depends primarily on the amount of coronal dentine available to assist in retention of the core, or, more exactly, an assessment of the quantity of sound coronal dentine that will remain following subsequent preparation for the indirect restoration. It is of interest that the amount of residual coronal dentine is often overestimated in the clinical setting[15].

Teeth requiring endodontic treatment have typically lost tooth structure (due to previous restorations and/or current caries): further loss of coronal dentine is necessary for endodontic access. As a result, there is often a lack of coronal dentine in which to prepare retentive features without compromising the strength of the remaining tooth structure. Nayyar and his co-workers described a technique whereby 2–3 mm of the coronal root filling is removed and an amalgam core placed to fill not only the coronal preparation, but also to fill the pulp chamber and extend into the roots[16]. Utilisation of the radicular portion of the tooth in this way provides good retention and resistance without the need to remove any more coronal tooth structure (Fig. 4.2). In the initial report, a very high success rate was reported.

This technique has been widely adopted and is also suitable for premolars as well as molars. Although it is usual to remove root-filling material from the coronal aspect of the root, in situations in which there is a large pulp chamber, extension of the amalgam into this space alone is sufficient. A core of this type will function well even when as little as one sound cusp remains and careful application of this technique can overcome problems related to limited retention of a direct core, while reducing the need for placement of an intra-radicular post and associated problems.

The main disadvantage of this technique is the difficulty of endodontic retreatment and the lack of any 'sealing' material between the root filling and the coronal restoration. The latter problem may be overcome if the technique is used with resin-modified glass-ionomer cement (RmGIC) as the core material, though a significant amount of coronal dentine must remain, as RmGIC is a weaker material and less suitable for use as a structural core.

If there is little remaining coronal dentine, then further retention for the core will need to be provided by the placement of an intra-radicular post. If some coronal dentine remains to provide some support, then a direct post in conjunction with a corono-radicular direct core should be placed. If very little coronal dentine remains then a cast post (indirectly constructed) should be provided. If a cast post is to be provided and more than one canal needs to be utilised to provide retention, as the canals are likely to be divergent, the core should be constructed in more than one piece (i.e. two or three, depending on how many intra-radicular posts are placed). Such a core is termed a 'split core'.

Intra-radicular posts

Historically it was understood that the placement of an intra-radicular post would reinforce the root and provide greater resistance to root fracture. Clinical studies have not shown reduction in fracture incidence by the placement of a post in pulpless teeth[10]; the bulk of remaining tooth structure rather than the presence of a post is important in providing resistance to fracture. The only exception to this is when a tooth has a very large canal space with thin root dentine walls at risk of fracture. Such a situation may typically arise in an upper incisor that became non-vital at a young age (typically due to trauma). The radicular dentine will be thin with a very large pulp space. It is possible that bonding techniques may allow for reinforcement for the root via placement of a low viscosity resin composite into the root with a light-transmitting intra-radicular post to allow for light-activated polymerisation of the resin composite to the full depth[17]. Although evidence for this is limited at present, it would seem to be a useful technique to reduce the potential for fracture of such teeth.

From available evidence it would appear that the only true indication for post placement in a tooth is to retain a core, more specifically:

- To retain a restoration when a lack of coronal tooth structure remains following root canal treatment. This lack of tooth structure would not enable satisfactory resistance or retentive form for a direct or indirect restoration without the placement of a post in order to retain a core.
- There is insufficient crown tissue left on a vital tooth to accommodate placement of a core (to support a crown). In such cases elective root treatment may be undertaken.

The term 'post-crown' is often used but perhaps 'post-retained core' is more appropriate.

Design requirements

Length

There is a direct relationship between post length and retention and in addition, the post must also be long enough to minimise internal stresses on the root. The exact dimensions of the ideal post have been considered in detail and these include:

- Equal to the length of the clinical crown[18,19]
- Half the length of the root[20]
- Longer than the final clinical crown[8]
- Midway between the apex and the height of the alveolar crest[21]
- Leaving 3–5 mm of root filling material[22]

While a disparity of opinions exists as to the length of post preparation, most investigators and clinicians agree that the post length must not interfere with the apical seal. Microleakage is considerably reduced if an excess of 4 mm of gutta-percha remains in the canal apical to the post[23,24].

Diameter

With respect to retention, diameter is not as important as post length with little or no increase in retention seen with increasing diameter. Post diameter should therefore not be increased in the hope of gaining retention but should solely be dictated by the physical properties of the post and canal morphology, in order to avoid removing an excess of sound tooth structure. Increasing the diameter unnecessarily weakens the remaining root and may predispose it to fracture.

Shape

Posts may be generally classified as tapered or parallel, threaded or non-threaded and with a variety of surface finishes. The post shape is an important factor in determining retention and stress distribution, and selection of post type is usually dictated by the clinical situation.

With respect to retention, tapered posts usually fare poorly; the greater the taper, the lower the retention. Due to the tapered design, these posts allow cement to flow and vent easily and hence perform favourably during cementation and before loading (as shown in photoelastic stress studies). However, during loading tapered posts demonstrate unfavourable stress distribution compared with parallel-sided posts[25], and are more likely to split the root due to wedging forces. Parallel-sided posts offer increased retention compared with tapered posts along with a more favourable stress distribution pattern on loading.

To alleviate hydrostatic pressure during cementation, cylindrical posts usually incorporate vents along their long axes. The resistance of cylindrical posts to torsional/rotational forces is low and hence whenever possible an anti-rotational feature should be included in the final post-core unit to improve resistance to these forces. A circular cross-sectional configuration of the prepared post space will not offer any significant resistance to rotation of the post, thus the normal eccentricity of the coronal portions of the canal should be accentuated to provide an anti-rotational feature. This may also act as a positive seat for the core at the coronal portion of the canal, thus preventing over seating and wedging within the root that could lead to vertical fracture.

Indirectly constructed intra-radicular posts are made from a replica or 'pattern' of the desired shape: this pattern may be custom made or constructed from preformed shapes. Custom posts are essentially posts made from a pattern of a freehand preparation of the canal space: this pattern is usually made indirectly on a cast (obtained from an impression of the preparation) but may be made directly in the mouth. Preformed shapes usually entail the use of a drill and matching post components. Such components may consist of 'blanks' used for impression taking, burnout patterns for construction of a pattern (either indirectly on a model or directly in the mouth) or may be prefabricated posts with a core either built up directly or a core cast onto the prefabricated post.

Surface finish

The threaded or screw post has been in use for the longest time[26,27]. Although increased retention is provided, care must be taken during insertion to avoid fracture of the root or post. Photoelastic studies have demonstrated high levels of residual stress with threaded posts in both loaded and unloaded states, and as such the increased retention afforded by use of threaded posts must be weighed against the potential for creating stress fracture of roots. Some studies have shown that posts with larger threads are less passive and such posts, especially if tapered, are more likely to be involved in root fractures[28,29].

The provision of serrations or roughening can increase the surface area of a post. Smooth posts demonstrate the lowest retentive values, while sandblasting smooth surfaces doubles their retentive value. The retentive value of smooth and sandblasted posts can be further increased by the addition of circumferential grooves, but such features may weaken the post itself.

Post material

Custom cast metal posts (type III yellow gold, base metal alloys or silver–palladium alloys) are the only universal way of achieving accurate adaptation to all root canal configurations, but as discussed above are not as retentive as parallel posts. Prefabricated post systems may utilise a burnout replica to construct a one-piece cast post and core or a wrought post onto which a core is cast. A wrought post is stronger than a cast post for a given diameter. However, wrought posts with cast-on cores are not consistently more resistant to fracture[30]. The strength advantage afforded by wrought gold is lost during casting; however a complete casting with fewer voids is more likely, especially with smaller diameters. The use of differing metals in such a situation offers the potential for corrosion and this may even lead to root fracture due to build up of pressure from corrosion products, especially if the post contains tin[31]. Wrought posts are also generally more expensive.

Direct intra-radicular posts are designed to be cemented into the tooth and a core built up intra-orally. Prefabricated wrought metal posts offer the advantage of superior strength compared with cast posts, particularly in diameters less than 1.5 mm, and they are also clinically convenient. As well as wrought gold, direct posts may be composed of titanium, stainless steel or newer materials such as fibre posts (posts with a resin matrix and carbon or quartz fibre) or ceramic.

A post fabricated from carbon-fibre reinforced epoxy resin became commercially available in 1992[32], and several fibre posts are now available, with quartz fibres being the most common. It is claimed that the physical properties of such posts are similar to that of dentine, although it has been suggested that the flexibility of the post *in situ* will not match that of the root, even if the elastic modulus is the same, due to the influence of the cement layer and core[33]. There also remains disagreement as to whether a stiffer post leads to more even distribution of stress or whether a post with low stiffness is preferred[34].

Increased longevity of the restoration is claimed due to the decrease in stress concentration[35], though there is no clinical evidence to support this statement. There are a number of large studies showing a reduction in incidence of root fracture when fibre posts are compared with more rigid posts[36–38] and thus it is wise to consider placement of a fibre post to retain a core in situations in which the root is at significant risk of fracture (e.g. a short root, short post and thin radicular dentine). However, there are few well controlled clinical studies and no reliable randomised controlled trials[39], though this is an area of research interest at present and more data may soon be available.

In response to the need for a post possessing optical properties compatible with an all-ceramic crown, an all-ceramic post has been developed. The post is made from zirconium polycrystals and has a high flexural strength and fracture toughness. Although designed for use with a composite core, a technique has been described to combine the post with a pressed glass core. Due to the brittle nature of these posts, they are extremely difficult to remove.

Choice of direct or indirect post-retained core

As with all indirect techniques, an indirect post will require an unimpeded path of insertion with no undercuts. In some situations in which a reasonable amount of dentine remains, placement of a direct post and direct core material (amalgam, resin composite etc.) will avoid unnecessary removal of sound tooth structure. When little

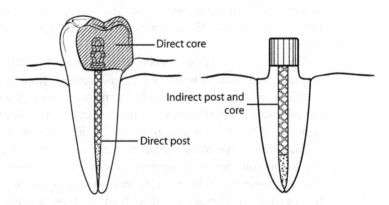

Fig. 4.3 Direct and indirect intra-radicular posts.

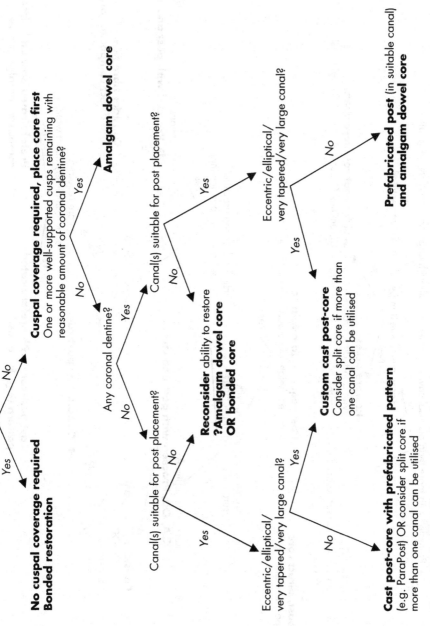

Fig. 4.4 Flow chart for restoration of molar teeth.

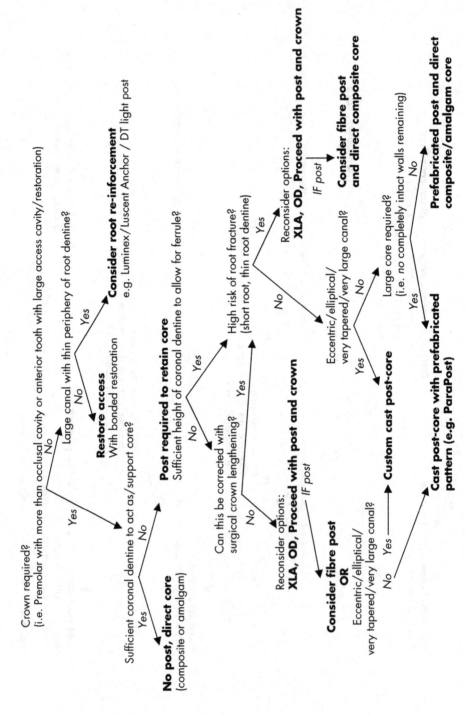

Fig. 4.5 Flow chart for restoration of premolar and anterior teeth (XLA = extraction, OD = over denture).

coronal dentine remains to provide strength and aid in retention of a core, then an indirect post with integral core is indicated (Fig. 4.3). In all cases, it is essential that the margin of the subsequent indirect restoration passes beyond the junction of the core and tooth, i.e. a ferrule is present (see Chapter 5).

The above principles for restoration of root-filled teeth are summarised in the flow diagrams in Figs 4.4 and 4.5.

REFERENCES

1. Andreasen J., Andreasen F.M., Bakland L. and Flores M. *Traumatic Dental Injuries: A Manual*, 2nd edn. Oxford, Blackwell Munksgaard, 2003.
2. Andreasen F.M. Transient root resorption after dental trauma: the clinician's dilemma. *J Esthet Restor Dent*, 2003; **15**: 80–92.
3. McNab S., Battistutta D., Taverne A. and Symons A.L. External apical root resorption following orthodontic treatment. *Angle Orthod*, 2000; **70**: 227–32.
4. Wedenberg C. and Lindskog S. Macrophage colonization of infected and non-infected dental tissues *in vitro*. *Scand J Dent Res*, 1986; **94**: 311–19.
5. Cvek M. Treatment of non-vital permanent incisors with calcium hydroxide. II. Effect on external root resorption in luxated teeth compared with effect of root filling with gutta percha. A follow-up. *Odontol Rev*, 1973; **24**: 343–54.
6. Abou-Rass M. The stressed pulp condition: an endodontic-restorative diagnostic concept. *J Prosthet Dent*, 1982; **48**: 264–7.
7. Reuter J.E. and Brose M.O. Failures in full crown retained dental bridges. *Br Dent J*, 1984; **157**: 61–3.
8. Guzy G.E. and Nicholls J.I. *In vitro* comparison of intact endodontically treated teeth with and without Endopost reinforcement. *J Prosthet Dent*, 1979; **42**: 39–44.
9. Sorensen J.A. and Martinoff J.T. Endodontically treated teeth as abutments. *J Prosthet Dent*, 1985; **53**: 631–6.
10. Sorensen J.A. and Martinoff J.T. Intracoronal reinforcement and coronal coverage: a study of endodontically treated teeth. *J Prosthet Dent*, 1984; **51**: 780–4.
11. Ray H.A. and Trope M. Periapical status of endodontically treated teeth in relation to the technical quality of the root filling and the coronal restoration. *Int Endod J*, 1995; **28**: 12–18.
12. Saunders W.P. and Saunders E.M. Coronal leakage as a cause of failure in root-canal therapy: a review. *Endod Dent Traumatol*, 1994; **10**: 105–8.
13. Hansen E.K. *In vivo* cusp fracture of endodontically treated premolars restored with MOD amalgam or MOD resin fillings. *Dent Mater*, 1988; **4**: 169–73.

14. Hansen E.K. and Asmussen E. *In vivo* fractures of endodontically treated posterior teeth restored with enamel-bonded resin. *Endod Dent Traumatol*, 1990; **6**: 218–25.

15. Bandlish R.B. Assessment of the amount of coronal dentine in root filled teeth. MSc thesis, University of London, 2001.

16. Nayyar A., Walton R.E. and Leonard L.A. An amalgam coronal-radicular dowel and core technique for endodontically treated posterior teeth. *J Prosthet Dent*, 1980; **43**: 511–15.

17. Lui J.L. Composite resin reinforcement of flared canals using light-transmitting plastic posts. *Quintessence Int*, 1994; **25**: 313–19.

18. Tidmarsh B.G. Restoration of endodontically treated teeth. *J Endod*, 1976; **2**: 374.

19. Colman H.L. Restoration of endodontically treated teeth. *Dent Clin North Am*, 1979; **23**: 647–51.

20. Goerig A.C. Restoration of teeth with subgingival and submucous fractures. *J Prosthet Dent*, 1975; **34**: 634.

21. Shadman H. and Azarmehr P. A direct technique for the fabrication of post and cores. *J Prosthet Dent*, 1975; **34**: 463–7.

22. Shillingburg H.T., Fischer B.W. and Dewhirst R.B. Restoration of the endodontically treated tooth. *J Prosthet Dent*, 1970; **24**: 401–7.

23. Neagley R.I. The effect of dowel preparation on the apical seal of endodontically treated teeth. *Oral Surg Oral Med Oral Pathol*, 1969; **28**: 739–45.

24. Zemener O. The effect of dowel preparation on the apical seal of endodontically treated teeth. *J Endod*, 1980; **6**: 687–90.

25. Henry D.J. Photoelastic analysis of post core restorations. *Aust Dent J*, 1977; **124**: 157–63.

26. Black G.V. A method of grafting artificial crowns on roots of teeth. *Mo Dent J*, 1869; **1**: 233–6.

27. Prothero J.H. *Prosthetic Dentistry*. Chicago, Medico-Dental Publishers, 1921.

28. Durney E.C. and Rosen H. Root fracture as a complication of post design and insertion: a laboratory study. *J Prosthet Dent*, 1977; **38**: 161–4.

29. Standlee J.P., Caputo A.A. and Holcomb J.P. The Dentatus screw: Comparative stress analysis with other endodontic dowel designs. *J Oral Rehabil*, 1982; **9**: 23–33.

30. Ryther J.S., Leary J.M., Aquilino S.A. and Diaz-Arnold A.M. Evaluation of the fracture resistance of a wrought post compared with completely cast post and cores. *J Prosthet Dent*, 1992; **68**: 443–8.

31. Rud J. and Omnell K.-A. Root fractures due to corrosion. *Scand J Dent Res*, 1970; **78**: 397–403.

32. Duret B., Reynaud M. and Duret F. A new concept of corono-radicular reconstruction: the Composipost (2). *Chir Dent Fr*, 1990; **60**: 69–77.

33. Morgano S.M. and Brackett S.B. Foundation restorations in fixed

prosthodontics: current knowledge and future needs. *J Prosthet Dent*, 1999; **82**: 643–57.

34. Asmussen E., Peutzfeldt A. and Heitmann T. Stiffness, elastic limit, and strength of newer types of endodontic posts. *J Dent*, 1999; **27**: 275–8.

35. Torbjorner A., Karlsson S., Syverud M. and Hensten-Petterson A. Carbon fiber reinforced root canal posts. Mechanical and cytotoxic properties. *Eur J Oral Sci*, 1996; **17**: 599–609.

36. Hedlund S.O., Johansson N.G. and Sjögren G. A retrospective study of prefabricated carbon fibre root canal posts. *J Oral Rehabil*, 2003; **30**: 1036–40.

37. Ferrari M., Vichi A. and Garcia-Godoy F. Clinical evaluation of fiber-reinforced epoxy resin posts and cast post and cores. *Am J Dent*, 2000; **13**: 15B–18B.

38. Ferrari M., Vichi A., Mannocci F. and Mason P.N. Retrospective study of the clinical performance of fiber posts. *Am J Dent*, 2000; **13**: 9B–13B.

39. Bateman G., Ricketts D.N. and Saunders W.P. Fibre-based post systems: a review. *Br Dent J*, 2003; **195**: 43–8; discussion 37.

5

INTRODUCTION AND INDICATIONS

An indirect restoration is any restoration that is fabricated extraorally. Although there are a few techniques that allow indirect restorations to be constructed at the chairside, the vast majority of indirect restorations are constructed in a dental laboratory. An indirect restoration will be then luted/cemented into/onto the tooth, in contrast with plastic restorative materials, which are packed directly into a preparation. As indirect restorations are rigid, in order to place them within or on the tooth they obviously require a preparation that is non-undercut (Fig. 5.1).

Indirect restorations may be broadly split into categories: intracoronal restorations that fit within the contours of a tooth (e.g. inlays, cast intra-radicular posts); extra-coronal restorations that cover the outer surface of a tooth to recreate the anatomic contours (e.g. full or

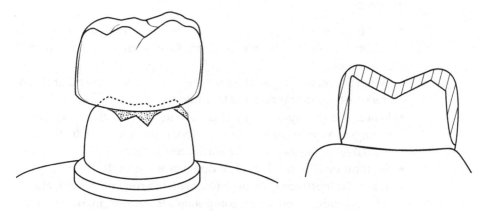

Fig. 5.1 Non-undercut preparation for indirect restoration (crown).

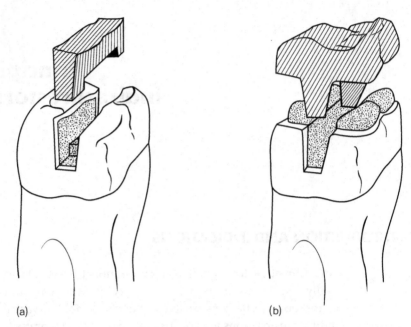

(a)   (b)

Fig. 5.2 Various types of indirect restoration. (a) Inlay, (b) onlay.

partial coverage crowns, veneers); and also those in-between restorations that cover part or all of the external surface of a tooth to recreate form and may also fit within the tooth (e.g. cuspal coverage inlay/onlay) (Fig. 5.2).

General indications

In general terms, indirect restorations are of benefit in the following situations:

- Large cavities/preparations – when correct anatomical form is difficult or impossible to reproduce with a directly placed restoration.
- When the remaining tooth structure is compromised and at risk of fracture (e.g. after root-canal treatment).
- When the restoration would be of such a size that alternative, stronger/more wear resistant materials are required (than those available for use as a directly placed restoration).
- Restoration of severely broken down or worn teeth.
- When the tooth has been prepared with instruments manufactured with matching pre-formed components (e.g. posts, inlay inserts).

Large cavities

Although teeth with large cavities involving multiple missing cusps may be restored with direct restorative materials, it is very difficult and technically demanding and errors often occur. Use of a direct restoration in this situation cannot always establish the contact point, and food packing and periodontal disease may result. In addition, recreation of correct occlusal morphology is very difficult with large, compound restorations. The use of an indirect restoration, such as an inlay will largely avoid these problems.

Risk of fracture

When there is a significant risk of tooth fracture steps should be taken to reduce the possibility of fracture occurring. As an aspect of their increased retention, bonded restorations provide support to weakened cusps[1,2]; however some doubt exists as to the long-term benefit. A more reliable method for preventing fracture in the long term is to provide a restoration with cuspal/occlusal coverage in order to protect the remaining tooth structure. Cuspal coverage can be provided by direct as well as indirect restorations[3] but, as indicated above, it is extremely demanding to place large restorations so that they fulfil all necessary criteria for a successful restoration with respect to recreation of form and occlusal contacts. Given a situation in which remaining cusps are thin and unsupported by a bulk of coronal dentine, an indirect restoration with cuspal coverage will reduce the risk of cusp fracture. Although this treatment will involve removal of some healthy tooth structure, it will act to preserve tooth substance by preventing tooth fracture.

In addition to teeth with unsupported cusps, root-treated teeth are also at risk of fracture. A consequence of root treatment of posterior teeth is that the remaining cusps are weakened owing to previous loss of tooth structure from earlier restorations and further loss of tooth structure due to the endodontic access. Posterior teeth provide the majority of support in the intercuspal position and any contact during excursive movement produces high lateral forces. As such, an endodontically treated tooth requiring more than an occlusal restoration has a significant risk of cusp fracture. A tooth with an intact marginal ridge has significantly more resistance to fracture than a tooth that has a cavity/preparation involving the marginal ridge. In order to prevent cusp fracture, in most endodontically treated posterior teeth it is sensible to consider provision of an indirect restoration that provides cuspal coverage.

Stronger materials

When any restoration is provided, the main factor to be considered for choice of material is the functional demands that will be placed on the restoration and the ability of available material to withstand these forces. Although amalgam has good compressive strength, it will not have sufficient mechanical properties for use in all situations, especially for very large restorations in posterior teeth subjected to high loads. It is often necessary to use an alternative material with more suitable properties, such as gold or ceramic (though ceramics are generally brittle and weak in tension).

Although there have been rapid and numerous advances in resin-based restorative materials for aesthetic restorations, the mechanical properties of these are still markedly inferior to that of amalgam. In situations in which demand for an aesthetic result is high and when direct resin-based restorations would not have sufficient strength or wear properties, an indirect restoration may be utilised. Resin composite inlay restorations made indirectly have the advantage that handling is easier and technique sensitivity is less with respect to control of poly-merisation shrinkage. In addition, it is thought that resin composite inlay restorations made indirectly have mechanical properties super-ior to similar directly placed materials, as they are polymerised under pressure and at a higher temperature so that the degree of con-version is higher. However, there is little clinical difference in wear[4]. Alternatively, ceramic inlays may be used, though these restorations must have enough bulk to provide sufficient strength. Resin com-posite and ceramic may also be used for cuspal coverage restorations.

Broken down and worn teeth

When there has been extensive loss of tooth structure due to caries, tooth or restoration fracture or due to other non-carious tooth tissue loss, it is often necessary to provide an indirect restoration.

In addition to the major examples described above, indirect restora-tions may also be used in a number of other situations:

- To restore teeth with structural defects, e.g. hypoplastic teeth.
- As part of a larger restoration/reconstruction, e.g. part of fixed bridge-work.

- For splinting, e.g. periodontally compromised teeth.
- For aesthetic improvement, to alter colour, shape, size or inclination of teeth.
- To alter occlusal relationships.

When deciding whether to provide an indirect restoration for a patient, the individual tooth should not be considered in isolation, but it is also essential to consider other factors that have a bearing on treatment:

- Patient motivation
- Oral hygiene status
- Periodontal condition
- The restorative state of the mouth
- Occlusal relationships
- Age of patient (size of pulp-space)

Once it has been decided that an indication exists for an indirect restoration, and that such an approach to treatment is suitable for that patient, then the type of core restoration and indirect restoration to be provided should be decided.

CORE RESTORATIONS

A core is the term used to describe the restoration that is placed in order to build up a broken down tooth before receiving an indirect restoration. In some cases it may not be necessary to place a separate core, but an indirect restoration may be constructed to replace all of the missing tooth structure. Typical examples of this include root-filled teeth in which an integral corono-radicular restoration and core may be placed[5], or for teeth that have suffered cusp fracture where placement of a traditional restoration would leave very little tooth structure (e.g. premolars with a previous mesio-occluso-distal restoration and one lost cusp, a 'one-piece' onlay may be the treatment of choice). However, for most teeth requiring an indirect restoration, a core restoration will need to be provided.

The exact nature of any particular core will depend on the degree to which the tooth in question is broken down and how much coronal dentine remains. When attempting to understand the rationale for choice of core restoration, it is helpful to consider the concept of extremes, from a simple space-filling core to a structural core (Fig. 5.3) and relate the different functions to the materials available.

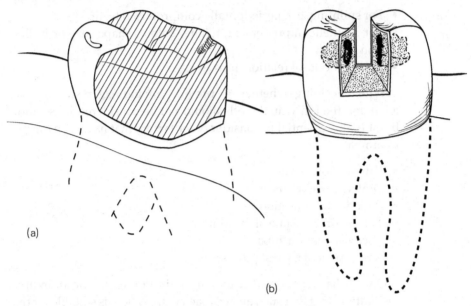

(a)

(b)

Fig. 5.3 Types of core restorations, (a) structural and (b) space-filling.

Space-filling core

When much coronal dentine remains, the role of a core is simply to fill out any undercuts and give an appropriate shape that will provide adequate retentive and resistance form (described later). The restorative material simply acts to prevent or 'block out' any undercuts to the path of insertion of the intended indirect restoration. This situation commonly arises when an intra-coronal restoration (i.e. an inlay) is planned to replace a previous direct restoration. The preparation will have to be modified to eliminate the undercuts; extending the preparation would be unnecessarily destructive compared with placement of a core material to block out the undercuts. Similarly, the same approach can be taken to give smooth axial walls when an extra-coronal restoration such as a full coverage crown is planned.

In the above example, the functional demands and stresses encountered by the core material will be minimal. The mechanical properties of a core material in this situation are not critical, and the material choice is largely determined by secondary factors such as ability to bond to tooth structure, cariostatic properties and ease of handling (e.g. command set).

Structural core

When a large amount of coronal dentine has been lost, it is more likely that an extra-coronal full-coverage restoration will be planned. The core material will replace a substantial part of the clinical crown and will form the bulk of the final preparation. In this case, the core material will be subjected to significant functional demands and stresses, particularly in molar teeth, and must therefore have adequate mechanical properties to resist these. Although a full-coverage crown may afford some protection to the core if the margins are extended gingivally beyond the core[6], this protection is limited. The strongest materials available at present are amalgam (for a direct core) or a cast metal such as gold (for an indirect core in an endodontically treated tooth).

Essentially, there are four types of direct core material available; amalgam, resin composite, glass ionomer or hybrid materials such as light-cured resin-modified glass-ionomer cement (RmGIC).

Amalgam

Amalgam has perhaps the best track record when used for substantial posterior core build-ups. Amalgam has good contrast with tooth substance and is easy to prepare. The long time to full set may predispose to early fracture, which is unfortunate, as the preparation cannot usually be prepared at the same visit, although newer high-copper amalgam alloys have high strength within a short time and may be prepared at the same visit after a short delay. The thermal expansion of amalgam is quite dissimilar to dentine, and this factor may predispose to failure after a period of time. In addition, amalgam cannot be bonded to tooth substance without resorting to proprietary products for amalgam bonding.

Resin composite

The use of resin composite as a core material has advantages and disadvantages. The composite does not require a two-visit crown preparation technique and, when necessary, the crown preparation can be commenced immediately. However, against this, the resin composite is difficult to prepare to the correct form because it may be difficult to differentiate between tooth tissue and core substance, though resin composites of contrasting colour are available. Light-cured resin composites should be used with caution, as full depth of cure may not be achieved in substantial core build-ups. Chemical-cure or dual-cure resin composites (the latter having the advantage of 'command set') have an advantage in that those portions of the material not exposed to the curing light will still undergo polymerisation due to the chemical cure. However, they may undergo increased discoloration (due to the tertiary amine activator[7]) compared with light-cured resin composites and thus should be used with caution in anterior teeth in which non-opaque aesthetic restorations are planned. Some resin composites are marketed specifically for core build-up, are coloured and have advantages over tooth-coloured composites. It has been suggested that because of water sorption and expansion, additional die relief should be provided during construction, or impression taking should be delayed after preparation to prevent discrepancy between the working die and the prepared tooth[8].

Glass ionomers and resin-modified glass-ionomer cement

Traditional glass-ionomer cements are only suitable for use as a space-filling core, where they will not be subjected to any stresses, as they are inherently weak materials. Several glass-ionomer materials are marketed specifically for use as a core build-up material such as RmGIC. They bond to dentine, release fluoride, have comparable thermal behaviour to dentine, can be made a contrasting colour to tooth (e.g. blue) and are easy to prepare, although the long-term behaviour of these materials is not well documented. Water sorption and expansion are higher with these materials than with resin composites and, for this reason, after preparation there should be a delay before impression taking. At present, their use as a structural core may be questionable. However they may eventually become the materials of choice with further developments.

Choice of core material

The choice of core material depends on several clinical variables. The role of the core material with regard to a space-filling or functional role is critical and the degree to which the core will be subjected to stress and the amount of bracing provided by remaining coronal dentine should be considered when selecting the material. Amalgam alloy should not be used beneath anterior full-veneer crown restorations as corrosion products from the amalgam core may stain the dentine peripheral to the restoration and result in poor aesthetics.

Similarly, an amalgam core underneath a three-quarter crown may shine through the remaining tooth and be unaesthetic.

Restoration of the endodontically treated tooth is covered in detail in Chapter 4, though points of particular relevance are repeated here. In most situations the general principles above apply. When little tooth structure remains it is usual to place a post-retained core, although molar teeth may successfully be restored with an amalgam dowel core (Nayyar core). If a direct intra-radicular post has been placed in order to retain a core, then care should be taken to ensure that the properties of the core material are not mismatched to those of the post (e.g. avoid glass-ionomer cement or resin-composite cores with metal intra-radicular posts), although some studies suggest that fibre posts (with a relatively low modulus of elasticity) perform better with a rigid metal core[9].

In general terms, when there is sufficient coronal dentine remaining to provide some support to the core material, then resin-based restorative materials are the core materials of choice. However, for a tooth that has lost much coronal tooth structure then a stronger core material (amalgam or cast metal if root treated) should be placed.

PRINCIPLES OF PREPARATION FOR INDIRECT RESTORATIONS

The general principles that apply when preparing and restoring any tooth have been covered in detail in the section on direct restorations. These principles are those guiding ideals that determine the rationale for operative intervention and the final form of the preparation produced and shape of restoration. In general, principles that apply to all restorations have either a mechanical or a biological basis and include steps to achieve:

- Elimination of diseased tissue
- Preservation of tooth structure
- Restoration of form
- Occlusal stability
- Pulpal health
- Periodontal health
- Durability of tooth and restoration
- Acceptable aesthetics

A few of these principles, either directly or by extrapolation, have particular importance when applied to preparation of teeth for provision of indirect restorations[10]. These are:

- Preservation of tooth structure
- Retention and resistance form
- Marginal integrity
- Strength and structural durability
- Occlusal stability

The following arguments apply equally to extra-coronal and intra-coronal restorations, though for simplicity, the explanations refer mostly to extra-coronal restorations.

Preservation of tooth structure

The need to preserve tooth structure wherever possible is axiomatic. With regard to the reduction and loss of tooth structure required to place an indirect restoration, it is important to note that although destructive, the provision of an extra-coronal restoration may actually result in preservation of tooth substance in the long term – for example, posterior root-filled teeth have a much higher fracture rate compared with similar teeth that have been crowned. In other cases in which indirect restorations are planned for an improvement in aesthetics only, for example aesthetic veneers, then the 'cost' to the tooth must be weighed carefully against the perceived benefit. In determining the amount of removal of tooth structure for provision of an indirect restoration, there are three main considerations: the requirement for protection from fracture and wear, the pattern of tooth substance removal and the type of restoration to be provided.

Protection from fracture and wear

Restorations providing cuspal coverage provide preservation of tooth structure by protecting the remaining axial walls from stresses that may subsequently lead to fracture of weakened, susceptible cusps. Also, a well-made indirect restoration that can control loads on the tooth by maintaining stable occlusal contacts may minimise load and wear on the tooth and restoration itself. Intra-coronal restorations, such as inlays, may also provide a similar degree of protection if they are adhesively bonded to the tooth, though an inlay that spans from one proximal surface to the other (i.e. mesio-occluso-distal) will create a wedging effect that inherently predisposes the tooth to fracture.

Pattern of tooth substance removal

Reduction of tooth structure should be appropriate and yet not excessive. There needs to be sufficient reduction to provide enough space to accommodate the required thickness of restorative material without necessitating overcontouring of the restoration. If too much tooth structure is removed, the health of the tooth will be compromised. Reduction must be anatomical, that is the reduction planes should broadly follow the contours of the tooth (or planned final shape) – a flat over-reduced occlusal surface will shorten the preparation, reducing retention as well as reducing the resistance form (Fig. 5.4). Conversely, inadequate reduction in the occlusal grooves will not provide adequate space for good functional morphology. Also, a flat single plane of reduction on the axial portions of the tooth will remove more tooth substance than is necessary, and will result in an uneven space for the restorative material[11].

There should be greater tooth substance removal over the functional cusp (i.e. palatal maxillary cusps or buccal mandibular cusps). This is usually achieved by means of a wide bevel. If this is not done and the crown is constructed to a normal contour then the resulting restoration will be too thin in this area. If adequate bulk is provided by over-contouring the final restoration, then the occlusal contacts will be incorrect, either too high or result in interferences during excursive movements. In addition, a lack of a functional bevel leads to uneven and uncontrolled distribution of stress and tensile forces on the cement lute.

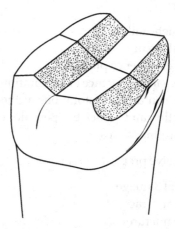

Fig. 5.4 Anatomical reduction.

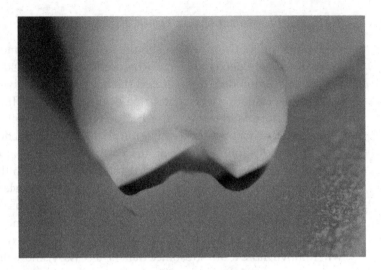

Fig. 5.5 Silicone index showing occlusal reduction.

Reduction is often overestimated. The use of depth grooves, or a bur tip of known diameter, is a useful aid[12], though a silicone index, either of the tooth before reduction or taken from a diagnostic wax-up of the intended shape, is the most reliable guide (Fig. 5.5). The most common errors are non-anatomical reduction or a lack of a functional bevel.

Poorly controlled reduction can lead to both technical and biological problems. Typical problems arising as a result of under-preparation include:

- Aesthetic failure
- Metal flexure
- Poor emergence profile
- Occlusal interference or perforation of the restoration
- Over-contoured restorations at the margin, which lead to plaque retention and associated periodontal problems and increased risk of marginal caries

Excessive preparation can lead to:

- Pulpal damage
- Ceramic fracture
- Core fracture

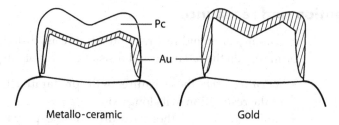

Pc

Au

Metallo-ceramic   Gold

Fig. 5.6 Reduction required for metallo-ceramic and cast metal restorations (Pc = porcelain, Au = gold).

Types of extra-coronal restoration

The type of extra-coronal restoration should be as conservative as possible while achieving the aims of treatment. Restorations may be simply categorised on the basis of the type of material to be used and on the amount of tooth covered (full or partial coverage).

The mechanical characteristics of the material chosen will dictate the amount of tooth substance removed. Extra-coronal restorations can be broadly categorised into three traditional categories, veneer metal (gold) restorations, all ceramic restorations and metallo-ceramic restorations.

The amount of reduction required will largely depend on the type of material to be used for the final restoration (Fig. 5.6), for example:

- Gold – 1 mm coverage occlusally with 1.5 mm over supporting cusp, may be 0.8 mm on palatal aspect of anterior teeth.
- Metallo-ceramic – 1.4 mm minimum on the facial surface of an anterior tooth.
- Ceramic – 1–1.5 mm on anterior teeth for traditional porcelain, less if the ceramic can be laminated to the tooth structure as with a resin-bonded crown, or up to 2.5 mm if a high-strength crystalline ceramic core is utilised.

An indirect restoration that covers all or most of the clinical crown is termed a full-coverage restoration, a partial-coverage restoration being one which leaves some of the clinical crown intact (e.g. onlay or capped cusp inlay, ³/₄ or ⁷/₈ crown, adhesive veneers). If retention (described later) can be maintained, intact surfaces of tooth structure should be saved and not removed for convenience or speed.

Retention and resistance

The ability of an indirect restoration to resist dislodging forces relies primarily on the retentive and resistance form of the preparation.

- *Retentive form* – those features of the preparation that resist removal of the restoration in its long axis.
- *Resistance form* – those features of the preparation that resist dislodgement due to forces outside the path of withdrawal of the restoration, i.e. lateral or rotational forces.

Resistance is probably the more important of the two. There exists a relationship between the two but this is not direct. The role of the cement lute should also be considered; traditional cements are strong in compression but weak in shear loads, therefore good resistance form (and retention) is necessary to minimise the shear loading on the luting cement. Adhesive cement lutes offer large increases in resistance and retention, but they should not be used simply to compensate for poor preparation. Both traditional and adhesive lutes may undergo fatigue failure, and uncertainty exists regarding the longevity of adhesive bonds. Therefore whichever type of lute is used, attention should still be given to achieving good retentive and resistance form.

Retention

Retention is primarily a surface area effect, depending on:

- Height of preparation
- Diameter
- Surface texture
- Taper

Of these, taper is the most critical factor. Theoretically, the more nearly parallel the opposing walls of a preparation, the greater the retention[13]. In order to avoid production of undercuts and to allow seating of the crown, a slight taper is cut. Various suggestions have been made regarding optimal taper, commonly 6° (5–10°) is quoted, though higher figures are often given for molars. The rationale for this is that full seating of a restoration is more important than a tight casting for good retention[14] (due to the role of the cement lute) and long teeth may need a greater taper in order to allow seating of the final crown. Resistance and retention will be excellent with a long crown. Less taper should be produced on short teeth when retention and resistance will be poor. Despite these arguments, the use of die-spacer (to provide space for the cement lute) will largely reduce problems with seating of restorations. Also, in order to maximise retention, it would be wise to aim for near parallelism in all cases, especially as most clinicians underestimate the amount of taper that has been produced[15,16]. When aiming to achieve near-parallelism, it should be remembered that burs commonly used for tooth preparation are tapered and simply need to be held in the long axis of the preparation in order to produce a taper.

Resistance

In order to increase resistance to displacement due to lateral or rotational forces, the preparation requires minimal taper and also increased height. The increased height of preparation must have a constant diameter as parallel walls that are not on the same base do not provide stability (Fig. 5.7).

When the clinical crown is short, or it is not possible to obtain near parallelism, additional features such as grooves, slots or boxes can enhance the resistance form significantly by reducing the radius of rotation of the final crown[17]. These features should be prepared in the long axis of the preparation and not just placed in line with the axial wall. Axial grooves should, if possible, be placed into sound tissue of a cusp and not into core material, which may be inherently weak. There should be a definite wall perpendicular to the direction of the force in order to limit the freedom of displacement and provide adequate resistance. Axial grooves effectively improve the height:diameter ratio, and enhance retention as well as resistance.

In some situations even the use of additional features will not provide enough resistance and in such cases surgical crown lengthening may be utilised to increase the available clinical crown height. This scenario, where the need to create interocclusal space by preparation would result in short crowns with limited resistance, is discussed in Chapter 6.

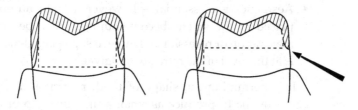

Fig. 5.7 Resistance provided by parallel walls at the same level.

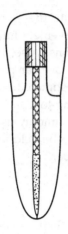

Fig. 5.8 Ferrule provided by extension of crown margins beyond core.

Marginal integrity

The margin of the restoration (or finishing line) is the area at which the restoration ends and presents a junction of restorative material and tooth substance at the tooth surface. Finishing lines should not routinely be placed subgingivally, but should be placed where they may be easily finished by the operator, cleaned by the patient and duplicated by the impression. They should be placed on sound tooth substance, not the core, as this would result in concentration of stress on the core and predisposition to failure. If possible, finishing lines should be placed on enamel (though it is common for margins to end on dentine or even cementum) and end 2 mm below the core[6] in order to support and protect the core through a ferrule effect (Fig 5.8). A ferrule will decrease the incidence of core fracture and will also decrease the incidence of root fracture with intra-radicular posts.

A sub-gingival margin may be inevitable when:

- Caries or a crack extends subgingivally.
- A restoration extends subgingivally.
- Extra axial length is required for retention.
- Aesthetics are essential – however a large number of margins placed in the sulcus become supragingival because of gingival maturation or recession. It has been suggested that ideal placement is at the level of the retracted gingivae[18].

In determining the shape of tooth reduction at the margin, the aim must be to produce as small a marginal gap or discrepancy as possible. Apart from the increased potential for caries with an open

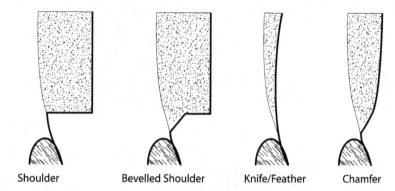

| Shoulder | Bevelled Shoulder | Knife/Feather | Chamfer |

Fig. 5.9 Margin configurations.

margin, larger marginal gaps may lead to periodontal problems and increased bone loss[19,20]. It is common in general engineering to utilise the principle of a slip joint; if the restoration has an acute edge at the margin, the marginal gap will be minimal even when a restoration fails to seat fully, i.e. the full occlusal discrepancy is not reflected at the margin. Production of such a 'slip joint' is not without problems, and for this reason a number of margin designs, suitable for varying applications, may be produced (Fig. 5.9). The margin design aims to achieve minimal marginal discrepancies while considering factors such as the mechanical properties of the material to be used and ease of construction.

Feather edge

The feather edge is the closest to a slip-joint that can be produced. It results in an acute angle of metal at the margin so that any failure to seat occlusally is not reflected totally at the margin. The feather edge margin is only applicable for a cast metal restoration, which is strong in thin section and may be burnished. However, feather-edge finishing lines should not be used as:

- They do not provide a definitive finishing line for the dentist.
- They do not provide a definitive finishing line for the technician.
- The axial wall of the casting may lack rigidity due to the fine edge of metal.
- The restoration margin may be overcontoured as a compromise to provide definition and rigidity.

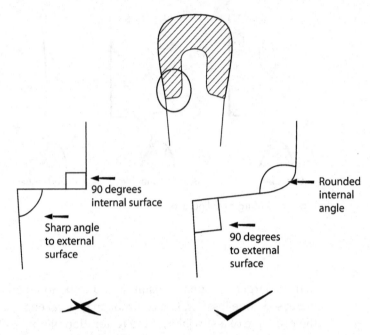

Fig. 5.10 Detail of shoulder margin.

Shoulder

The shoulder (or heavy chamfer/rounded shoulder) is the margin type necessary for ceramic restorations due to their brittleness and liability to fracture other than in compressive loads. The margin ensures that a relatively wide ledge provides support for the ceramic to resist occlusal forces and minimise tensile stresses that may lead to fracture of the ceramic. The shoulder should be produced to form a 90° angle to the external preparation margin. The sharp, 90° internal line angle classically associated with this margin concentrates stress in the tooth and sharp edges of ceramic may be rounded during firing, resulting in reduced accuracy of fit. Thus this internal angle should be rounded (Fig. 5.10), hence terms such as heavy chamfer (though this may lead to confusion) and rounded shoulder are used.

The shoulder is generally not used for metal restorations as it will not provide the acute margin that, as described above, will minimise marginal gaps and allow the margin to be burnished. However, it has been suggested that the shoulder finish may, in fact, give less of a marginal gap than a feather edge despite the theoretical advantages of the 'slip-joint'[21]. This is primarily because of problems of expressing cement lute from inside the casting during seating, which is more difficult with increased speed of seating and an acute margin. A more horizontal margin will result in the marginal gap not closing until the casting is nearly fully seated. A casting made to fit a shoulder margin may therefore have better fit, but the shoulder preparation is more destructive than other margin types and should be avoided when possible.

Chamfer

A chamfer is a compromise between the feather and shoulder finish. The chamfered finishing line is that of choice for metal restorations. It provides an acute margin, which is desirable, yet allows for escape of the cement lute. It also results in a restoration that has adequate axial bulk to provide rigidity without the need to overcontour and without being overly destructive of tooth substance, as a chamfer is more conservative of tooth substance than is the shoulder, as less axial reduction is necessary. It also exhibits the least stress (the underlying cement will have less likelihood of failure) and is readily identified on the die.

Bevelled shoulder

A shoulder with a bevel can also be used to create an acute edge of metal at the margin but should not be used routinely for veneer metal crowns as in this scenario it is unnecessarily destructive. It can however be used as a finishing line for partial coverage restorations.

Structural durability

For an indirect restoration to be able to withstand functional forces, it must be rigid enough to resist flexure and thick enough to resist wear and fracture. Rigidity is especially important at the margins of restorations – if the axial portion is too thin, for example with an acute feather-edge finishing line, the restoration is at risk of deformation and may result in breakage of the cement lute. The restoration must also be thick enough to resist wear and when reducing a tooth, sufficient reduction must be made in order for the restoration to have adequate thickness, for example, 1 mm occlusal and 1.5 mm functional cusp coverage for gold, 1.75–2 mm for a metallo-ceramic crown.

Structural durability requires control of stresses[22]. Chamfers concentrate stresses less than shoulders. As mentioned previously, when a shoulder is to be used, the junction between the base of the axial wall and the gingival margin of the preparation should be rounded to minimise stress in this area. Rounding of the reduced cusps, near parallel preparations and multiple point contacts on the final occlusion also reduce stress.

Occlusal stability

As discussed in Chapter 1, any new restoration must be in harmony with the existing occlusion if this is satisfactory, but may be used to create a new occlusal relationship in situations when the existing pattern is not satisfactory. In order for this to be determined, pre-operative examination of the occlusion is obviously essential. This may involve the use of study models mounted with a face bow record on an articulator, especially if multiple units or units involving guiding surfaces are to be restored. Note must be taken of existing relationships, both static (intercuspal position) and excursive (canine guidance or group function, anterior guidance and the presence of excursive interferences or gross discrepancies in movement from a retruded position to the intercuspal position).

The new restoration should be constructed such that it has sufficient contacts with the opposing tooth/teeth to maintain a stable relationship, which will also depend upon the durability of the material from which it is constructed. In addition, if the restoration is to provide a guiding surface, then the nature of this guidance (for example, whether to copy or change the existing relationship) must be carefully planned before the preparation is commenced.

SUMMARY

Principles of preparation for indirect restorations

(1) Preservation of tooth structure
  - Protection from fracture and wear
  - Pattern of tooth substance removal
  - Type of restoration

(2) Retention and resistance
  - Retention
    — Height of preparation
    — Diameter
    — Surface texture
    — Taper
  - Resistance
    — Increased height
    — Reduced taper
    — Additional features

(3) Marginal integrity
  - Feather edge
  - Shoulder
  - Chamfer
  - Bevelled shoulder

(4) Strength and structural durability

(5) Occlusal stability

REFERENCES

---

1. Hansen E.K. and Asmussen E. *In vivo* fractures of endodontically treated posterior teeth restored with enamel-bonded resin. *Endod Dent Traumatol*, 1990; **6**: 218–25.
2. Mach Z., Regent J., Staninec M., Mrklas L. and Setcos J.C. The integrity of bonded amalgam restorations: a clinical evaluation after five years. *J Am Dent Assoc*, 2002; **133**: 460–7.
3. Doukoudakis S. and Doukoudakis A. Amalgam onlay restoration. *J Prosthet Dent*, 1991; **66**: 493–7.
4. Wendt S.L., Jr and Leinfelder K.F. Clinical evaluation of a heat-treated resin composite inlay: 3-year results. *Am J Dent*, 1992; **5**: 258–62.

5. Nayyar A., Walton R.E. and Leonard L.A. An amalgam coronal-radicular dowel and core technique for endodontically treated posterior teeth. *J Prosthet Dent*, 1980; **43**: 511–15.

6. Hoag E.P. and Dwyer T.G. A comparative evaluation of three post and core techniques. *J Prosthet Dent*, 1982; **47**: 177–81.

7. Ranby B. and Rabek J.F. Photodegradation, photo-oxidation and photostabilization of polymers: principles and applications. London, Wiley, 1975, pp. 241–3.

8. Oliva R.A. and Lowe J.A. Dimensional stability of composite used as a core material. *J Prosthet Dent*, 1986; **56**: 554–61.

9. King P.A., Setchell D.J. and Rees J.S. Clinical evaluation of a carbon fibre reinforced carbon endodontic post. *J Oral Rehabil*, 2003; **30**: 785–9.

10. Shillingburg H.T.J., Hobo S., Whitsett L.D., Jacobi R. and Brackett S.E. *Fundamentals of Fixed Prosthodontics*, 3rd edn. Chicago, Quintessence, 1997.

11. Aminian A. and Brunton P.A. A comparison of the depths produced using three different tooth preparation techniques. *J Prosthet Dent*, 2003; **89**: 19–22.

12. Brunton P.A., Aminian A. and Wilson N.H.F. Tooth preparation techniques for porcelain laminate veneers. *Br Dent J*, 2000; **189**: 260–2.

13. Jorgensen K.D. The relationship between retention and convergence angle in cemented veneer crowns. *Acta Odontol Scand*, 1955; **13**: 35–40.

14. Lorey R.E. and Myers G.E. The retentive qualities of bridge retainers. *J Am Dent Assoc*, 1968; **76**: 568–72.

15. Smith C.T., Gary J.J., Conkin J.E. and Franks H.L. Effective taper criterion for the full veneer crown preparation in preclinical prosthodontics. *J Prosthodont*, 1999; **8**: 196–200.

16. Nordlander J., Weir D., Stoffer W. and Ochi S. The taper of clinical preparations for fixed prosthodontics. *J Prosthet Dent*, 1988; **60**: 148–51.

17. Owen C.P. Retention and resistance in preparations for extracoronal restorations. Part II: Practical and clinical studies. *J Prosthet Dent*, 1986; **56**: 148–53.

18. Silness J. Periodontal conditions in patients treated with dental bridges. 3. The relationship between the location of the crown margin and the periodontal condition. *J Periodontal Res*, 1970; **5**: 225–9.

19. Silness J. Periodontal conditions in patients treated with dental bridges. 2. The influence of full and partial crowns on plaque accumulation, development of gingivitis and pocket formation. *J Periodontal Res*, 1970; **5**: 219–24.

20. Felton D.A., Kanoy B.E., Bayne S.C. and Wirthman G.P. Effect of *in vivo* crown margin discrepancies on periodontal health. *J Prosthet Dent*, 1991; **65**: 357–64.

21. Ostlund L.E. Cavity design and mathematics: their effect on gaps at the margins of cast restorations. *Oper Dent*, 1985; **10**: 122–37.

22. Craig R.G. and Farah J.W. Stress analysis and design of single restorations and fixed bridges. *Oral Sci Rev*, 1977; **10**: 45–74.

Indirect restorations – further considerations

6

MATERIAL TYPE

Essentially the primary factors influencing choice of restorative material are the mechanical and aesthetic properties of the available materials in relation to the clinical situation. The main important factors to consider are:

- Functional demands
- Space
- Aesthetics
- Patient wishes

Functional demands

The need to consider the functional demands on a restoration is mainly related to the potential for wear and/or fracture, and the ability of the available materials to resist these. The principal influences on functional demand are mainly related to the occlusal relationships (see Chapter 1). More specifically, these are:

- *Nature of movement from the intercuspal position (ICP) during excursive movements.* If teeth are separated as soon as an excursive movement begins (termed immediate disclusion or point centric), then the degree to which opposing teeth will rub over each other is minimised, hence reducing the propensity for wear. If there is some 'rubbing' contact between opposing teeth before disclusion (delayed disclusion or long/wide centric), then it would be wise to choose materials for the functional surfaces that are more able to resist this wear, i.e. metal.

- *Nature and type of tooth contact during excursive movements.* If only a pair of canines contact during excursive movement and all other teeth are separated (i.e. they disclude) they 'provide the guidance', and this relationship is termed canine guidance. If more teeth are involved in guidance, this relationship is termed 'group function'. It is widely thought that canine guidance will result in less wear of the posterior teeth and will also protect the posterior teeth from lateral loads. Although little evidence exists to support this view, separation of the posterior teeth during excursive movements will allow more flexibility in choice of material used to restore the posterior teeth. Similarly, contacts between opposing teeth on the non-working side may place high lateral loads on teeth. If such teeth are to be restored, and these contacts cannot be removed, then a material that is better able to withstand these lateral loads should be used, i.e. metal.

- *Parafunctional habits.* Opposing teeth are normally only in contact for a short time, typically during mastication and swallowing. Habits such as bruxism/grinding or clenching will dramatically increase the contact time and hence increase the propensity for wear. In addition, as well as an increase in contact time, higher loads are usually placed on the teeth. In a patient who has a bruxist or clenching habit, it would be wise to carefully consider the likelihood of fracture before placing all ceramic restorations. Generally in these situations, restorations are more likely to last if functional and guiding surfaces are in metal.

- *Opposing dentition.* When planning a restoration, the potential for the opposing dentition to become worn or to wear the restoration should be considered. In general terms 'matching' materials are best if the opposing teeth have previously been restored. Metal (especially gold) is the least abrasive to opposing tooth structure[1], though in most situations ceramics may be employed, provided there is not a high potential for wear, as discussed above. Obviously, if there is no opposing tooth contact then there will be no (or minimal) load on the restoration and no concerns regarding wear and the choice of restorative material may be made with impunity. The ability to achieve stable occlusal contacts with available materials should also be considered. In situations in which many occlusal surfaces are to be restored, then multiple contacts will need to be provided in order to achieve or maintain occlusal stability. Ideally, this should not influence material choice. However multiple contacts are hard to obtain with ceramic restoration and require the skills of a highly competent technician.

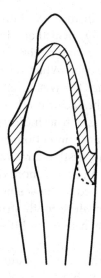

Fig. 6.1 Preparation modification with labial metal collar for long teeth. (Dotted line shows preparation for ceramic margin.)

Space

Obviously, interocclusal space (in the intercuspal position) is required for the placement of any restorative material. Ceramic requires more bulk (and therefore space) than metal (gold), which is strong in thinner sections. Interocclusal space is routinely provided by preparation of the tooth and removal of tooth structure. Generally, the degree to which reduction can be performed occlusally without compromising retention and resistance or the health of the tooth will determine whether it will be possible to have ceramic on the occlusal surface. Problems arsing from limited crown height are dealt with later.

There is also a relationship between crown height and choice of material, especially with anterior teeth. Restorations on 'long' teeth, when the margin has to be placed gingivally, may have to have a metal margin otherwise preparation for a ceramic margin may encroach on pulp space (Fig. 6.1). This will also result in a better contour and emergence profile and lessen the chances of problems associated with plaque retention. This also applies to bulbous molar teeth when the margin often has to be placed on radicular dentine.

Aesthetics and patient wishes

There is an increasing demand for aesthetic restorations. The need for an aesthetically acceptable restoration should never be overlooked. In general, better aesthetics are possible with all ceramic restorations owing to better optical properties and translucency. Although liked by some, metal restorations are obviously unaesthetic but in some situations (e.g. limited space for the restorative material or need for a strong material) then no alternative exists. When deciding what material to use, it can be debated whether the wishes of the patient are the most important, or only important, factor if other factors are equivocal. In situations in which there is a true indication for the use of (unaesthetic) metal and the primary intention of treatment is to provide a functional rather than an aesthetic result, then this should be explained. All-ceramic restorations are more destructive. However, if sufficient space can be provided for an aesthetic ceramic restoration without undue removal of healthy tooth structure, and wear and fracture are not a concern, then there is little argument against providing such treatment.

In summary, when considering material selection, although various materials are available, the choice is basically between metal (gold), ceramic or a combination of both (metallo-ceramic).

Cast metal (gold) is regarded by many to be the most satisfactory extra-coronal restorative material, has a hardness similar to enamel, does not creep intra-orally, can be cast accurately, and wax carving allows good detail and contour. It can be used in thin section with fine margins and hence requires only a small amount of reduction. Gold is not aesthetic, though it is liked by some.

All-ceramic restorations are the most aesthetic yet are brittle and liable to fracture, especially in thin sections, thus more bulk is needed than for gold. Generally, ceramic restorations are not strong enough to be used alone for posterior teeth or bridgework, though restorations made with a high-strength crystalline core show promise for use as single units or short-span bridges where there is adequate coronal height for the extra bulk of connector[2,3]. Cracks may arise from micropores on the surface, which may then open in tension or bending, especially if not supported, and this influences margin design. Dental porcelains are harder than enamel and if unglazed may abrade tooth surface.

Metallo-ceramic restorations (typically for full coverage crowns) allow good strength along with good aesthetics but require much more tooth reduction than alternatives in order to provide space for the metal substructure and sufficient ceramic for an aesthetic result. Although ceramic is frequently used for the functional surface, ideally this should be in metal in order to preserve tooth structure (no need for extra reduction to accommodate the ceramic). A metal occlusal surface will also avoid the overcontoured, wider occlusal table often present with ceramic occlusal surfaces and thus reduce the possibility of producing a non-working interference and give a better functional surface that is less likely to abrade the opposing dentition.

INTRA/EXTRA-CORONAL RESTORATION

The choice between provision of an intra-coronal or extra-coronal restoration is usually straightforward. When an indirect restoration is indicated owing to problems in achieving a functional result with direct materials or when a stronger material than those available for direct restoration is needed, then an intra-coronal restoration is an obvious choice. However, this presupposes that the axial walls of the tooth are intact and are not prone to fracture. If the axial walls of a tooth are substantially broken down and in need of restoration, then an extra-coronal restoration would be better suited.

There are, however, situations in which the decision is less straightforward, for example large preparations that span from one proximal area to another, leaving thin and tall unsupported cusps. Placement of an intra-coronal restoration would result in wedging forces and predispose the remaining cusps to fracture. Although a bonded restoration could be placed in the hope that the bond would protect the cusps, this is not as reliable as providing cuspal coverage, i.e. a reinforcing extra-coronal element to the restoration. This may simply be done by placing an inlay that also overlays the occlusal surface and a little of the axial surface (Fig. 5.2). However, as the size of such restorations increases, the difficulty also increases and placement of restorations with both intra-coronal and extra-coronal elements becomes more problematic – excess expansion of the investment during casting affects the fit of intra-coronal elements and conversely too little expansion of investment or shrinkage of resin composite/ceramic will affect the fit of extra-coronal elements. In many cases provision of an extra-coronal restoration is more reliable, particularly if the preparation is complex.

PARTIAL-COVERAGE RESTORATIONS

Advantages of partial-coverage restorations include:

* Preservation of tooth structure due to part of the clinical crown not being reduced, though the requirement for additional features for

retention/resistance (described on p. 145) may demand more removal. However, this is likely to be at the expense of the core rather than healthy tooth structure.

- Natural landmarks more likely to be preserved and this may aid preparation and also aid laboratory construction (easier to visualise the emergence profile).
- Margins are more likely to be supragingival and hence it will be easier to obtain an impression and to finish/polish margins as well as perform maintenance.
- Better seating on cementation as the axial walls are not covered to such an extent, thus expression of excess cement is easier than with full-coverage restorations.
- Access for pulp testing is maintained.
- Maintained vitality more likely.

Disadvantages of partial-coverage restorations include:

- Limited retention and resistance form.
- Aesthetic limitations.
- Technically demanding.

TEMPORISATION

Rationale for use of temporary restorations

Once a tooth has been prepared for an indirect restoration, there is usually a delay during which the restoration is constructed in the laboratory. During this period it is essential to provide a temporary restoration in order to:

- Protect the exposed dentine, prevent postoperative sensitivity and provide pulp protection to maintain tooth health.
- Protect the remaining tooth structure and preparation from risk of fracture.
- Maintain space by providing stable occlusal contacts to prevent overeruption of the prepared or opposing tooth.
- Maintain space by providing interproximal contacts with adjacent teeth to prevent drifting of the prepared or adjacent teeth.
- Be well fitting to allow good plaque control and prevent overgrowth of gingival soft tissues, which may otherwise prevent seating of the final restoration.
- Maintain aesthetics.

Provisional restorations

In most cases in which an indirect restoration is to be provided, the final result is easily determined and the treatment relatively straightforward. In these situations, a temporary restoration need only fulfil the roles listed above. There are, however, situations in which determination of the final shape of the definitive restoration is not as easy, or when there are complicating factors, such as where the existing aesthetics or occlusal scheme is to be altered. In such cases, temporary restorations may also have other roles and it is useful to make the distinction between simple temporary restorations, which fulfil the roles above, and provisional restorations, which serve additional functions.

Provisional restorations may be used to:

- Trial a planned tooth shape
- Delay provision of definitive restoration

The great value of a temporary restoration is that it can be used to 'try out' a planned shape before construction of the definitive restoration. Such ability is invaluable when considerable alterations are made to aesthetics, as modifications may be made to temporary restorations to achieve an acceptable result. Trial of the form of the restoration is also essential when significant changes are being made to occlusal relationships. Should the temporary restorations be uncomfortable, or suffer repeated fracture or loss of cementation then the planned occlusal scheme should be reviewed. Similarly, changes to palatal contour and incisal length of anterior teeth may affect phonetics, and this may also be assessed.

Temporary restorations may also be used to delay provision of the definitive restoration and can be placed for longer than the short time usually required. This is useful when periodontal health is compromised (e.g. to allow for resolution of gingival inflammation when previous restorations have had poor margins) or to allow for complete healing when surgical procedures have been performed. Long-term temporary restorations may also be useful for intermediate restoration of teeth with questionable prognosis before construction of definitive restorations (e.g. to allow for peri-radicular healing of endodontically treated teeth).

Temporisation of inlay preparations

In most cases inlay preparations are relatively small and simply require the preparation to be filled with a material that can be removed easily. Proprietary materials specifically intended for this purpose are available, consisting of a resin-based material that is simply placed in the preparation and polymerised with a light-curing unit. These materials do not need to be cemented and are easily removed when needed. Although very convenient, these have disadvantages of needing adequate bulk and also occlusal stability is difficult to achieve – occlusal contacts must be present on the unprepared tooth as the materials are hard to shape and relatively soft. When these materials cannot be used, a custom-made temporary inlay may be constructed from direct resin composite (placed in the preparation with a separating medium, polymerised, removed and then cemented), although the presence of any undercuts in the preparation will prove disastrous as the composite will then need to be removed with a bur with subsequent risk of further loss of tooth structure and damage to the preparation. An alternative is simply to fill the preparation with a traditional cement (e.g. zinc polycarboxylate). Great care is required to remove these cements without damage to the tooth/preparation.

Types of temporary crown

Temporary crowns may be made using a prefabricated crown or may be custom made; the latter can be constructed chairside or indirectly. The choice of material is largely determined by the aesthetic and mechanical properties.

Prefabricated crowns

A wide variety of prefabricated crowns is available and these vary in quality and anatomic form – some being so poorly shaped that they would not be able to fulfil the roles of a temporary restoration. Prefabricated crowns may be made from metal (typically aluminium or stainless steel) for use posteriorly or from plastic (typically from polycarbonate) for use when aesthetics are more important. A prefabricated crown is essentially a shell that can be trimmed to follow the contours of the margin and further adjusted to achieve adequate occlusal contacts. Although these types of temporary crown may be trimmed to fit and filled with a bulk of cement, a much better result is obtained if the shell is relined with a resin material. This will result in better stability of the temporary restoration as well as vastly improved marginal fit. Both metal and plastic shells may be relined in this way, although some roughening of the internal surface is often required to allow the relining resin to be retained within the shell.

Custom-made temporary crowns

Rather than relying on the shape of prefabricated crowns, a temporary crown may be custom-made for each patient. When a temporary crown is to be used as a provisional restoration or when multiple units are being restored, then this is the method of choice. Custom temporary crowns may be made at the chairside or indirectly.

Chairside custom temporary crowns are made using a pattern or matrix of the required tooth shape. When only a few crowns are required and the tooth shape before preparation is an acceptable form, then this matrix may be made from the teeth at the start of treatment. When the existing teeth are not of acceptable form or when a provisional restoration is required, this matrix should be constructed from a diagnostic wax-up of the intended result. Alginate or silicone putty may be used to form the matrix (Fig. 6.2), or a vacuum-formed stent may be constructed from a stone duplicate of the diagnostic wax-up. A variety of resin materials may be used to construct the temporary crown. Polymethylmethacrylate or higher molecular weight methacrylates may be used and can be easily modified to result in very well-fitting restorations; however these materials are

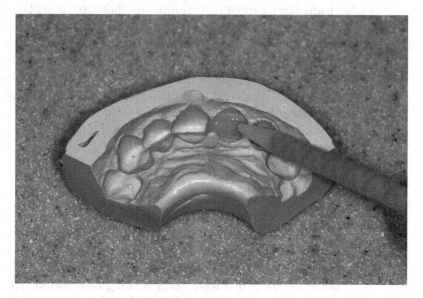

Fig. 6.2 Matrix being filled for custom temporary.

difficult to handle and have an exothermic setting reaction and a large amount of excess monomer, both of which may be injurious to the health of the tooth when in contact with freshly cut dentine[4]. Proprietary materials containing bis-acrylates are also available for construction of temporary restorations. These materials have low shrinkage, so result in a good marginal fit, have a low exothermic reaction on setting and have less potential for pulpal irritation[5,6]. Additions to these materials are possible with resin composite (due to similar chemistry) though this is not as easy or reliable as additions to methacrylates. When using these materials, care should be taken to ensure that the resin does not flow into undercuts (or is removed before set) so that the temporary restoration may be removed. The temporary restoration is then trimmed and polished before cementation.

When time allows, custom temporary restorations may be made indirectly. An impression is taken of the prepared teeth, and is poured in a quick-setting stone. The temporary restorations are then constructed as above using a matrix. The main advantage of this method is that acrylic resins may be used without the worry of irritant effects of heat and monomer. The acrylic can be cured under heat and pressure to give a strong restoration. This method is useful when multiple indirect restorations are required, and these can be more reliably made in this way, although the length of the patient's appointment is increased and on-site laboratory support is required.

As well as the relatively quick procedures outlined above, provisional restorations that are intricate, that need to be placed for a long time or may be subjected to large stresses (e.g. extensive temporary restoration in a bruxist), may be made indirectly in a similar manner to definitive restorations. These may be made from heat-cured acrylic, resin composite or one of these materials in combination with a metal substructure (e.g. cast gold or silver). These methods require much more time for construction and in such cases it would be usual to provide a short-term temporary restoration, while the provisional restoration is constructed.

Temporary cementation

There are several materials available for temporary cementation. Essentially any temporary cement must be weak enough to allow easy removal of the temporary restoration and residual cement from the preparation, yet strong enough to retain the temporary restoration while the definitive restoration is being constructed. The choice of material is based on the retention available in that a preparation with poor retentive form will require the use of a stronger temporary cement. In addition, the constituents of the temporary cement should not interfere with the final cementation.

It is often suggested that eugenol-containing temporary cements may reduce bond strengths obtained with definitive resin-based cement[7,8] (the eugenol acts as a plasticiser and weakens the bond) though this has been questioned[9,10]. Various eugenol-free temporary cements are available for routine use, and it is uncommon to require a stronger cement. A close fitting rigid temporary restoration (e.g. metal and acrylic provisional restoration) may be very difficult to remove if these cements are used and most can be modified by the addition of a small amount of petroleum jelly.

IMPRESSION TAKING

When an indirect restoration is provided, it is usual to take an impression of the prepared tooth and use this impression to create a model on which the restoration is constructed. Obviously, the restoration can only be as accurate as the impression, and the influence of the gingival tissues and choice of material for this impression are critical.

Gingival management

Periodontal disease should be controlled such that the state of the periodontal tissues is optimised before any procedure and maintained thereafter. Untreated periodontal disease compromises success of restorative treatment and poor restorative treatment leads to adverse effects on the periodontium. The fit and quality of restorations are of paramount importance – defective margins are directly related to the severity of periodontal disease[11,12]. When margins of a preparation are above the level of the gingivae, impression taking is relatively straightforward. However due to the very nature of teeth that require such restorations having had multiple previous restorations, it is usual that the margins are close to, at, or even below the level of the gingivae. In this situation, obtaining an accurate recording of the margin of the preparation becomes more difficult and not only is it necessary to record the margin, but it is also necessary to record unprepared tooth beyond the margin in order that the restoration can be constructed with the correct emergence profile. In order to achieve this, the gingival tissues require careful handling and will need to be retracted, i.e. moved away from the margin while the preparation is taken, and gingival exudates or haemorrhage must be controlled. There are several ways in which this may be achieved, including use of:

- Physical gingival retraction
- Chemical agents
- Electrosurgery
- Rotary gingival curettage

Physical gingival retraction

Physical retraction of the gingivae for impression taking is primarily achieved with retraction cord. This is a fine cord that is placed into the gingival sulcus and left *in situ* for a short time in order to ease the marginal gingival tissues away from the preparation (Figs 6.3, 6.4). Braided and knitted cords are available, knitted cords having the advantage that they are less likely to unravel. Other materials are also available to retract gingival tissues physically, including synthetic polymers (Merocel)[13] and expanding synthetic materials[14].

The length of time that the cord is left in place is important; too short and the gingivae will not be adequately retracted, but too long may result in damage to the sulcular epithelium[15]. Only light pressure

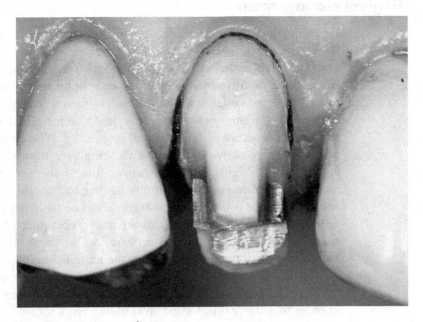

Fig. 6.3 Retraction cord *in situ*.

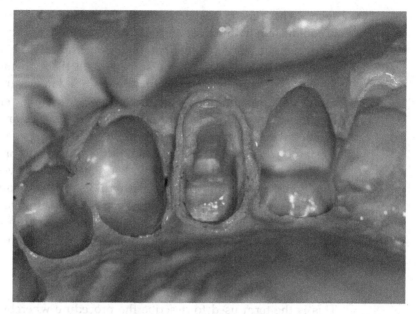

Fig. 6.4 Working impression.

should be used to place the cord as excess packing force may push the cord beyond the periodontal attachment into supra-alveolar connective tissue which will be too deep to retract the gingivae and may result in trauma. It may be advantageous to place two cords, with a fine cord placed first. This will remain in place during impression taking. This has the advantage of controlling gingival exudates or haemorrhage that may persist when a single cord is used; however great care must be taken not to insert the cord too deep and to remember to remove the cord after the recording of the impression.

When the impression material is ready, the cord may be removed or left *in situ* if the margin is clearly visible. Care should be taken if the cord is removed as the sulcular epithelium may be damaged, especially if the cord is removed dry. Trauma should be avoided as it may lead to haemorrhage from the gingival tissues, thus making it impossible to obtain an accurate impression of the margin. In addition, significant trauma to the gingival tissues may result in apical migration of the gingival margin and can lead to unaesthetic visible margins.

Chemical agents

Several chemical agents are available for control of gingival exudates and haemorrhage, and are essentially either vasoactive or clotting agents. These chemical agents may be used alone or may also be used in conjunction with retraction cord. Many chemical agents have been used, including alum, sympathomimetics such as racemic adrenaline, aluminium chloride and ferric sulphate. All these chemicals have the potential to traumatise gingival tissues[16] and may cause necrosis of sulcular epithelium. Adrenaline has possible systemic effects, and has been shown to cause cardiovascular disturbances and is better avoided when halothane is being administered during general anaesthesia or when an adverse reaction with concurrent conditions or medication may occur (e.g. beta-blockers, antihypertensives, tricyclic antidepressants, uncontrolled hyperthyroidism, etc.) Agents that control exudates by promoting clotting, such as ferric sulphate, appear to be safe in small quantities, though these agents can cause staining of the tooth and gingival tissues and should be used with care.

Electrosurgery

This is the term used to describe the procedure whereby high frequency electrical energy is used to cut and coagulate soft tissues. An active electrode tip directs energy, and various tips are available. Use of a narrow tip leads to localised tissue dehydration and disintegration (cutting), whereas a broad tip spreads current and can be used to produce coagulation. A passive electrode (often termed a grounding plate) is a large plate placed remote from the operating site and allows the current to pass through the patient's body from the active electrode. Most electrosurgery units are capable of producing a variety of waveforms. A fully rectified and filtered waveform results in good cutting and minimal shrinkage but poor haemostasis (usually labelled 'cut'). A fully rectified, not filtered waveform will give good haemostasis as well as cutting tissue with little shrinkage (usually labelled 'cut/coag') and is versatile. A partially rectified waveform will give inefficient cutting and causes tissue shrinkage but is useful with a ball-ended electrode to control haemorrhage (usually labelled 'coag').

Electrosurgery can be used for gingival retraction and for access to subgingival margins, though as with most techniques there are a number of advantages and disadvantages:

Advantages:

- Easy retraction of multiple abutments
- Clear vision of finishing line
- Increased bulk of impression material

- Decreased operative time
- Haemostasis
- Predictable healing, little discomfort

Disadvantages:

- Odour/taste (high volume suction is required)
- Technique sensitive
- Little tactile feedback
- Should not be used on or near patients with pacemakers
- Must not be used near flammable gases!
- May cause trauma to the tooth[17] or adjacent supporting tissues with poor technique
- Equipment cost
- Should not be used with topical local anaesthetic (which is flammable)

Rotary gingival curettage

Rotary gingival curettage is the term used to describe the simultaneous preparation of the tooth and removal of the inner part of the sulcal epithelium. There is little or no tactile feedback during this procedure, which is obviously traumatic to the gingivae and therefore leads to apical relocation of marginal tissues. In addition the frank haemorrhage that occurs with this technique requires control in order to take an impression, which can usually only be achieved with a material that is hydrophilic, such as reversible hydrocolloid. Visualisation of the preparation margin is also difficult and uncertain. This technique should not be used routinely and is largely historical.

METHODS OF CONSTRUCTION

There are a number of ways in which indirect restorations, constructed extra-orally, may be made. The most common methods utilise an indirect pattern, though computer-aided design and computer-aided machining techniques (CAD/CAM) may be employed, as may a direct pattern.

Indirect pattern

Once a preparation has been completed, an impression is taken to record fine detail. An impression of the opposing arch is also taken.

The impression is disinfected and sent to the dental laboratory where a gypsum-based plaster is poured into the impression to make a model. The restoration is either made directly on a model of the tooth formed from phosphate-bonded gypsum (termed a refractory die) for resin composite or ceramic, or is made on a model formed from die-stone (Type IV) for metal restorations (by investing and casting a wax pattern). Due to the number of separate steps involved in this process and the potential for inaccuracies at several stages (e.g. distortion of the impression, expansion of gypsum products) it is technique sensitive. However, this method of construction is well established and each stage well understood, and as the pattern for the restoration and/or restoration itself is made in controlled conditions, a high level of accuracy can be achieved.

Direct pattern

An alternative to forming a pattern in the laboratory from a replica of the preparation is to form a pattern directly intra-orally from the tooth itself. This is usually only appropriate for metal restorations, when a pattern is made either in casting wax or acrylic. This method has obvious advantages in that as fewer stages are involved compared with an indirect pattern, then the potential for errors is small and accuracy of fit is high. However, the pattern should be invested as soon as possible after it has been formed to avoid distortion. This method is technically demanding to perform, especially if occlusal surfaces are involved and is therefore only suitable for small restorations. It is particularly suited for creating patterns for post-retained cores.

Computer-aided design and computer-aided machining techniques (CAD/CAM)

Several propriety systems exist for creation of ceramic restorations at the chairside. A system-specific intra-oral camera captures an image of the cavity or preparation (often termed a 'three-dimensional optical impression'). Most software packages then allow some modification of the image (e.g. identification of margins). The planned shape of the final restoration is then machined from a block of ceramic.

This method has the obvious advantage of avoiding multiple visits. Also the restorations produced are strong when compared with traditional dental porcelains, as the restorations can be milled from a block of industrially sintered ceramic, which will have fewer flaws.

Although the laboratory costs are eliminated, CAD/CAM systems require a large initial outlay. In addition the occlusal surface of restorations is not as accurately produced compared with laboratory restorations, and some systems require the occlusal surface to be shaped intra-orally by the operator. A further disadvantage is that aesthetics are limited because of the small range of available colours and monochromacity, as the restoration is machined from a single block.

LIMITED RESISTANCE AND RETENTION

When a preparation has limited retentive and resistance form, there are a number of steps that may be taken to reduce the potential loss of the restoration. These include limiting influence of lateral forces with additional preparation features, utilising adhesive luting cements and increasing crown height.

Additional preparation features

If a groove is placed into the axial wall(s) of a preparation, this will reduce the moment arm of the force that acts to dislodge a restoration about a point of rotation. Shortening this radius of rotation will increase the resistance form of a preparation. This effect can be visualised as a short tapered preparation in which the placement of a groove results in the restoration 'engaging' against a wall of the preparation at an earlier point, so that a larger portion of the preparation acts to resist the rotational force. This is shown schematically in Fig. 6.5. Multiple parallel grooves will significantly limit the path of withdrawal and increase both resistance and retention of the final restoration.

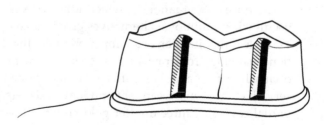

Fig. 6.5 Grooves providing additional resistance form.

Adhesively retained restorations

Retention of a restoration is markedly influenced by the type of luting cement, and restorations cemented with an adhesive lute require much higher forces to dislodge them. Advances in adhesive techniques have added another mode of treatment in addition to more conventional techniques. Resin-based composite materials may be reliably bonded with similar resin-based luting cements, which may also be for luting ceramic restorations following etching and silane treatment of the ceramic fitting surface. Base metals may be bonded to tooth structure with bi-functional polymeric resins, for example phosphonated esters of Bis-GMA (bisphenol A-glycidyl methacrylate), and gold may also be reliably bonded to tooth structure following heat-treatment[18] (to produce a chemically active oxide layer on the fitting surface of the restoration). Although long-term studies are limited, there is clinical evidence that indirect restorations bonded to tooth structure survive well in the oral environment[19].

Adhesively bonded restorations may permit preservation of tooth structure when compared with more destructive traditional options. For example, the use of bonded restorations to prevent cusp fracture rather than reducing and overlaying cusps. Adhesive techniques are also very useful when retention is at a premium and when a traditional preparation would involve removal of a large amount of healthy tooth structure or may result in exposure of the pulp.

Adhesively retained restorations often prove useful in restoring defects caused by tooth wear/non-carious tooth tissue loss (NCTTL). Anterior NCTTL typically occurs on palatal surfaces and these may be restored with cobalt–chromium or gold veneers cemented with resin. This technique is relatively easy. Maximal coverage up to and including the incisal edge is provided to increase retention and aid placement. Thin metal palatal veneers can also be used in conjunction with labial resin composite to increase tooth length. Posterior NCTTL can also be restored with adhesively retained gold castings, which are useful when space is limited.

There are also situations in which adhesive restorations may prove useful when traditional alternatives give limited options. A common example is the situation of an upper premolar that has a large restoration spanning from one proximal surface to the other across the occlusal surface and has suffered a cusp fracture. The most conservative traditional treatment option would be to place a core and a partial-coverage, three-quarter gold crown. However, the visibility of gold is not very aesthetic and is often unacceptable to patients. The traditional aesthetic alternative would be to place a full-coverage metallo-ceramic crown with ceramic on the visible parts of the tooth; however this would require removal of a significant amount of tooth structure. The use of an adhesive restoration would allow for an aesthetic onlay/inlay to be directly bonded to the remaining tooth structure with little additional preparation.

Increasing crown height

The height of a preparation may be simply increased by placing the margin more gingivally, perhaps subgingivally. However, this may predispose to periodontal problems. Increasing periodontal problems may present when margins move from being supragingival to crestal to subgingival. With deeper margins, there is likely to be more inflammation, increased pocket depth and possibly loss of attachment[20]. Margins should ideally be no more than 0.5 mm subgingivally in order to keep clear of the attachment complex. If margins impinge on the epithelial attachment or connective tissue, then inflammation and potential periodontal problems result.

If margins are subgingival, or when there is a need to increase the clinical crown height, then surgical crown lengthening may be considered. In healthy tissues there is a consistent relationship between the crest of alveolar bone, the length of epithelial attachment and sulcus depth. This relationship has been termed 'biological width' and is the minimum width at the gingival sulcus required to maintain a normal gingival attachment[21]. Removal of soft tissue alone would not result in this relationship and thus apical movement of the entire attachment apparatus is necessary, requiring removal of bone in order to maintain health.

When aesthetics are critical, for example in the anterior segment of a patient with a high smile line, a contralateral procedure may be necessary to retain symmetry. Also, if a single tooth requires crown lengthening and supporting bone is removed from that tooth only, the gingivae may not rest more apically but may 'bridge' the gap: thus a procedure on a single tooth may involve bone removal around adjacent teeth.

CREATION OF INTEROCCLUSAL SPACE

In order to place an indirect restoration, particularly an extra-coronal restoration, then the tooth usually has to be reduced to provide sufficient interocclusal clearance for the restorative material (i.e. space between the tooth requiring a restoration and opposing teeth when the remaining teeth are together in the intercuspal position). This space in the intercuspal position is required at the fossae regions and for the supporting cusps. Although it is usually necessary to reduce the non-functional cusp, this is not universally so. Space for the non-functional cusps (remember their position in excursion) is determined by the anterior and posterior determinants of the functional occlusion (see Chapter 1) that in turn determine the degree of separation of opposing teeth during excursive movements. These are:

- Condylar guidance
- Anterior guidance
- Curves of Spee, Wilson, Monson
- Occlusal plane angle
- Non-working interferences (especially if on the tooth to be restored)
- Premature contact (and slide from RCP to ICP on tooth to be restored)

In some situations, it may be possible to encroach on the space available during disclusion of opposing teeth rather than reducing a non-functional cusp, though great care is required not to introduce a non-working interference or to produce an unaesthetic restoration and this approach alone is seldom enough to overcome space problems.

In some situations in which space is limited, thin adhesively retained metal-cast restorations may prove useful, as described previously. In other situations, this approach cannot be used, for example when preparation would result in exposure of the pulp, when only very short preparations are possible with little retention or when space for the restorative material is at a premium. In these situations it is usually necessary to create more interocclusal space for the restorative material without unnecessary tooth reduction. This may be achieved through orthodontic movement of the tooth to be restored or by increasing the occlusal vertical dimension.

Orthodontic movement

Formal orthodontics may be a useful adjunct, either involving movement of individual or multiple teeth (e.g. uprighting molars or flattening the curve of Spee). However, in many cases localised axial tooth movement may be simply and easily performed. This method was first described by Dahl[22,23], who utilised a removable appliance that increased load onto selected anterior teeth resulting in axial movement. The space obtained is a combination of intrusion of the teeth with the 'Dahl appliance' and extrusion of the remaining teeth, the pattern of movement differs between individual patients, though age appears to be a factor with intrusion predominating in older patients[24].

The technique, often termed the 'Dahl principle'[25], has been developed and techniques involving indirect metal splints cemented onto teeth[24] and individual restorations (usually resin composite) placed 'high' have been described[26]. The use of individual build-ups on anterior teeth rather than splinting teeth together may cause splaying and labial movement, though this does not appear to be a problem in most cases. Space for restorations needed in a localised area only can be created, for example by providing interocclusal space anteriorly by moving all six teeth, and the principle may also be utilised to move individual teeth, for example to correct over eruption. There is an increasing trend to cement definitive anterior restorations in 'high' and rely on this movement. Although this approach is very convenient, this technique offers less control over occlusal relationships and in many instances it is prudent to create space and then provide the definitive restorations to an exact and planned occlusal relationship. This technique may be employed posteriorly or anteriorly and is particularly useful for managing cases involving tooth wear.

Increasing the occlusal vertical dimension

Increasing the occlusal vertical dimension (OVD) and providing restorations without occlusal reduction will allow restorations to be placed with less need for tooth substance removal. However, this approach is more clinically demanding, is complex and requires a very compliant patient. The dentition will normally need to be restored at the retruded axis position (RAP), hence a period of stabilisation splint wear will be required (which will also aid in treatment by providing stability). In addition, a major disadvantage of this approach is that multiple restorations will be required in order to re-establish occlusal contact between all teeth.

In many cases in which multiple teeth require restoration and space is at a premium, for example tooth wear, a combination of approaches is required. Also, when there are very short clinical crowns, surgical crown lengthening may be performed to increase clinical crown height and increase retention, as described previously.

LIMITATIONS OF INDIRECT RESTORATIONS

Indirect restorations typically have a longer lifespan than similar direct restorations[27]. However, it is a common misconception that once an indirect restoration is placed then the tooth does not require any care. In fact, the opposite is true. Any indirect restoration will have a 'long' margin that is essentially its weak point with respect to caries. It is not uncommon for caries to progress rapidly along the margins of a restoration such as a crown and for this caries to go unnoticed for some time. Caries at the margins of indirect restorations is often not detected until it has progressed so far as to make further restoration of the tooth questionable at best, and often impossible. It is essential that follow-up and maintenance are provided for any restoration and especially for indirect restorations.

Provision of indirect restorations entails a significant increase in costs due to the extra time and need for multiple appointments and also the cost involved in production of the restoration. Although it would appear that indirect restorations are more expensive to provide than direct restorations, over a lifetime, this may not be the case as there will be fewer interventions due to the increased longevity of the restoration[28,29].

Without judicious application of the correct technique, indirect restorations may be harmful to the tooth. For example, an inlay that spans from one proximal surface to the other (i.e. mesio-occluso-distal) will inherently predispose the tooth to fracture owing to its wedging effect. It should also be remembered that many indirect restorations entail a 'cost' to the tooth due to the need for the removal of (often substantial) amounts of tooth structure and possible pulpal injury.

REFERENCES

1. Jagger D.C. and Harrison A. An *in vitro* investigation into the wear effects of selected restorative materials on enamel. *J Oral Rehabil*, 1995; **22**: 275–81.
2. Odman P. and Andersson B. Procera AllCeram crowns followed for 5 to 10.5 years: a prospective clinical study. *Int J Prosthodont*, 2001; **14**: 504–9.
3. Fischer H., Weber M. and Marx R. Lifetime prediction of all-ceramic bridges by computational methods. *J Dent Res*, 2003; **82**: 238–42.
4. Langeland K. and Langeland L.K. Pulp reactions to crown preparation, impression, temporary crown fixation, and permanent cementation. *J Prosthet Dent*, 1965; **15**: 129–43.

5. Fleisch L., Cleaton-Jones P., Forbes M., van Wyk J. and Fat C. Pulpal response to a bis-acryl-plastic (Protemp) temporary crown and bridge material. *J Oral Pathol*, 1984; **13**: 622–31.

6. Driscoll C.F., Woolsey G. and Ferguson W.M. Comparison of exothermic release during polymerization of four materials used to fabricate interim restorations. *J Prosthet Dent*, 1991; **65**: 504–6.

7. DeWald J.P., Moody C.R. and Ferracane J.L. Softening of composite resin by moisture and cements. *Quintessence Int*, 1988; **19**: 619–21.

8. Millstein P.L. and Nathanson D. Effects of temporary cementation on permanent cement retention to composite resin cores. *J Prosthet Dent*, 1992; **67**: 856–9.

9. Peutzfeldt A. and Asmussen E. Influence of eugenol-containing temporary cement on efficacy of dentin-bonding systems. *Eur J Oral Sci*, 1999; **107**: 65–9.

10. Ganss C. and Jung M. Effect of eugenol-containing temporary cements on bond strength of composite to dentin. *Oper Dent*, 1998; **23**: 55–62.

11. Silness J. Periodontal conditions in patients treated with dental bridges. *J Periodontal Res*, 1970; **5**: 60–8.

12. Padbury A., Jr, Eber R. and Wang H.L. Interactions between the gingiva and the margin of restorations. *J Clin Periodontol*, 2003; **30**: 379–85.

13. Ferrari M., Cagidiaco M.C. and Ercoli C. Tissue management with a new gingival retraction material: a preliminary clinical report. *J Prosthet Dent*, 1996; **75**: 242–7.

14. Shannon A. Expanded clinical uses of a novel tissue-retraction material. *Compend Contin Educ Dent*, 2002; **23**: 3–6.

15. Loe H. and Silness J. Tissue reactions to string packs used in fixed restorations. *J Prosthet Dent*, 1963; **13**: 318–23.

16. Kopac I., Sterle M. and Marion L. Electron microscopic analysis of the effects of chemical retraction agents on cultured rat keratinocytes. *J Prosthet Dent*, 2002; **87**: 51–6.

17. Spangberg L.S., Hellden L., Robertson P.B. and Levy B.M. Pulpal effects of electrosurgery involving based and unbased cervical amalgam restorations. *Oral Surg Oral Med Oral Pathol*, 1982; **54**: 678–85.

18. Eder A. and Wickens J. Surface treatment of gold alloys for resin adhesion. *Quintessence Int*, 1996; **27**: 35–40.

19. Djemal S., Setchell D., King P. and Wickens J. Long-term survival characteristics of 832 resin-retained bridges and splints provided in a post-graduate teaching hospital between 1978 and 1993. *J Oral Rehabil*, 1999; **26**: 302–20.

20. Silness J. Periodontal conditions in patients treated with dental bridges. 2. The influence of full and partial crowns on plaque accumulation, development of gingivitis and pocket formation. *J Periodontal Res*, 1970; **5**: 219–24.

21. Gargiulo A.W. Dimensions and relations of the dentogingival junction in humans. *J Periodontol*, 1961; **32**: 261–267.

22. Dahl B.L., Krogstad O. and Karlsen K. An alternative treatment in cases with advanced localized attrition. *J Oral Rehabil*, 1975; **2**: 209–14.

23. Dahl B.L. and Krogstad O. The effect of a partial bite raising splint on the occlusal face height. An x-ray cephalometric study in human adults. *Acta Odontol Scand*, 1982; **40**: 17–24.

24. Gough M.B. and Setchell D.J. A retrospective study of 50 treatments using an appliance to produce localised occlusal space by relative axial tooth movement. *Br Dent J*, 1999; **187**: 134–9.

25. Briggs P.F., Bishop K. and Djemal S. The clinical evolution of the 'Dahl Principle'. *Br Dent J*, 1997; **183**: 171–6.

26. Redman C.D., Hemmings K.W. and Good J.A. The survival and clinical performance of resin-based composite restorations used to treat localised anterior tooth wear. *Br Dent J*, 2003; **194**: 566–72.

27. NHS Centre for Reviews and Dissemination. *Undertaking Systematic Reviews of Research on Effectiveness: CRD's Guidance for Carrying Out or Commissioning Reviews*, 2nd edn. NHS Centre for Reviews and Dissemination, University of York, 2001.

28. Wilson N.H.F., Burke F.J. and Mjor I.A. Reasons for placement and replacement of restorations of direct restorative materials by a selected group of practitioners in the United Kingdom. *Quintessence Int*, 1997; **28**: 245–8.

29. Mjor I.A., Burke F.J. and Wilson N.H.F. The relative cost of different restorations in the UK. *Br Dent J*, 1997; **182**: 286–9.

Maintenance of the restored dentition 7

MAINTENANCE

It is a common public misconception that a restoration requires less care than a natural tooth; however the introduction of an interface between the restoration and tooth surface presents a 'weak-spot' that is prone to both biological and mechanical failure. It is important that for any intervention, a maintenance programme is developed for each patient to reduce future problems. Oral hygiene instruction and home care form major parts of a preventive programme for each patient, and can reduce the incidence of future disease[1].

Whenever any restorative intervention has been undertaken, there is an implication that disease (caries) or mechanical failure has occurred. To place a restoration without considering these factors will expose the restoration to an uncontrolled and unstable environment with an increased likelihood of failure. A correct diagnosis is essential before any treatment and in all cases, aetiological factors should be controlled as much as is possible.

For example, if mechanical failure has presented as multiple fractures of teeth or restorations, provision of an occlusal splint to control and distribute the excessive occlusal forces would be of benefit. Similarly, where failure is due to recurrent caries or there is a high caries risk, the importance of regular exposure to fluoride should be remembered and appropriate fluoride supplements (e.g. mouthwash) should be advised.

Although the above steps will help to avoid failure, deterioration of restorations is inevitable. All restorations will fail, i.e. dental restorations do not have infinite service life in normal clinical conditions. Survival time of simple restorations has been shown, in several surveys, to be of the order of 5–10 years[2–5]. With high quality treatment and a good preventive programme, then restorations may remain serviceable and functional for considerable periods of time. However, as failure is likely to occur at some point, regular review and an observant/aware patient will help to detect problems at an early stage when simple remedial treatment rather than extensive treatment may be performed. The recognition, management and replacement of dental restorations is therefore a routine component of the provision of continuing dental care.

FAILURE

Although there are many studies addressing failure/longevity of dental restorations, many of these do not provide useful information, as the definition of failure is often not given. There is variation between studies with regard to definition of failure with a variation from minor deterioration to a need for operative intervention or replacement of a restoration all being cited. The adoption of criteria for evaluation of dental restorations set by the United States Public Health Service (USHPS)[6] has helped to standardise assessment criteria, but there still exists a wide variation in the methodology of clinical trials available to support longevity figures for various types of restorations. Commonly identified risk factors[2,3,7,8] for increased likelihood of failure of a restoration include gender (higher failure in males), presence of occlusal contact (worse marginal deterioration), number of surfaces (three surface restorations have up to 1.8× risk of failure compared with two surface restorations) and operator (failure rates vary between operators with many failures being due to poor technique).

Recognition of failure

Failure of a restoration may take many forms and may be due to major defects (such as fracture and loss of a portion of the supporting tooth or restoration) or may be due to minor defects such as marginal deficiencies, staining or microleakage. When a restoration has failed, but does not involve loss of restoration or tooth bulk, it is unlikely that the failure will be noticed by the patient unless there are symptoms or there is a visible aesthetic problem. This is apparent for both direct and indirect restorations[9]. A delay in treatment of a failed restoration may result in further damage to the tooth or render repair impossible and as such it is important that an appropriate maintenance programme for a patient with a restored dentition includes frequent recall appointments, at which deterioration or failure can be recognised at an early stage by a clinician.

Most marginal defects are directly observable. In addition to clinical examination, radiographs are a useful adjunct to identify interproximal marginal defects/deficiencies or caries that may otherwise go unnoticed[10]. Also given the incidence of loss of vitality of teeth with indirect restorations, especially long-term[11], periapical radiographs may be useful to detect peri-radicular pathology.

It is easy to replace a failed restoration without considering the implications of failure, which are often underestimated. Situations such as sub-standard treatment, incorrect diagnosis (initially or of failure) or provision of restorations with a short life expectancy will all result in more frequent intervention. Quite simply, the implications of failure relate to cost, both in terms of economic implications as well as harm to the tooth.

Economics of failure

It is axiomatic that there is an economic cost implication in provision of any treatment, whether this cost is met by individual patients or is state funded. There are financial implications in treatment of failed restorations and also in preventing failure, and this should be transparent at the outset of treatment to both operator and patient. The relationship between initial cost and longevity is not always obvious, and in some cases a more costly initial treatment option may prove to be more cost effective in the long term[4].

Costs to the tooth

With any operative intervention there is a 'cost' to the tooth in terms of loss of tooth structure and trauma to the dentino-pulpal complex. This is true for any procedure, and loss of healthy tooth structure can be significant when restorations are removed for replacement, especially when tooth-coloured restorations are removed[12]. Two concepts of use are that of the 'life cycle' of a restored tooth, and that of the 'stressed pulp syndrome'[13]. The first describes the (sometimes inevitable) progression from a minimal intervention to a larger and larger restoration eventually necessitating an indirect restoration – emphasising the cumulative destructive nature of multiple interventions. The concept of a stressed pulp arises from the supposed healing of the dental pulp following trauma during an operative procedure. With each traumatic event, the pulp heals with a degree of tertiary dentine formation and fibrosis within the pulp. Successive interventions leave the pulpal tissues more fibrosed and less able to respond dynamically to trauma. Eventually, the pulp will be unable to withstand even a minor insult and may become non-vital with a relatively small intervention. These concepts suggest that whenever possible, the number of interventions during a tooth's life span should be minimised and each 'stage' of a tooth should be prolonged and interventions minimised in order to prolong the overall life of the tooth.

REPLACEMENT AND REPAIR OF RESTORATIONS

Failed or defective restorations that are associated with a clinically significant loss of function, tissue inflammation, or pulpal pathology should be replaced, adjusted or repaired (if possible), providing such treatment can be expected to overcome the problem. Surface quality deficiencies alone do not constitute an adequate reason for replacement[14]. It must be remembered that the cyclic replacement of restorations is associated with loss of tooth tissue due to progressive cavity/preparation enlargement and repeated insults to the pulp.

In recent years there has been a shift towards maintenance and repair[15], rather than the replacement of the deteriorating yet serviceable restorations in patients who maintain a good standard of oral hygiene. These patients with favourable oral environment and low caries risk should receive minimum intervention.

As a clinician, one must be able to:

- Diagnose a failed restoration.
- Analyse the reason for failure.
- Design the repaired/replacement restoration.
- Efficiently remove failed restorative material.
- Apply/insert corrected restoration.

Management decision

Although a fault may be identified, operative interference may not be warranted. A minor defect of a restoration margin with no signs of caries due to microleakage is a serviceable restoration. All operative interventions carry risk of additional damage to remaining natural tissues and intervening in a situation such as this will result in unwarranted removal of healthy tooth structure. Where minor defects have occurred, it is often possible to adjust local features and avoid radical reconstruction for example, clear occlusal interference and remove ledges from restorations or make minimal marginal additions.

When a fault is present but is localised to one region of the restoration, then consideration should be given to repairing rather than replacing the restoration, such that the intervention is minimised. Similarly, when caries is present adjacent to a restoration margin, then considering the lesion as a new/primary lesion and providing a localised repair will also act to preserve the health of the tooth. Although evidence for survival of repaired restorations is sparse, there are reports of good short-term survival rates[16,17]. When possible the observable defect should not only be corrected but preventive factors established to reduce the incidence of recurrent problems. When such additions/repairs can be made the new preparation should be designed to be as much as possible within the old restoration and shaped so that it will afford sufficient extension to:

- Eradicate the old defect.
- Permit adequate operative access when inserting the new restoration.
- Provide sufficient resistance and retention form to retain the new restoration.

Removal of an entire restoration that has a fault may be necessary; however such radical retreatment must be undertaken in the light of cost–benefit analysis, which includes the strategic value of the tooth and the anticipated service life of the new restoration. During the removal of the old restoration, sectioning of fragments of the restoration rather than removing every bit (with attendant problems of time, vibration, visibility and over-extension) will help to minimise the amount of healthy tooth structure lost. The failed restoration should be studied to identify effective planes of section, for example, across the isthmus of old compound amalgams followed by sagittal sectioning of both key and box, thereby allowing the remaining pieces to 'fall into' the body of the preparation for convenient extrication. Care should be taken when prising any remaining adherent pieces of the restoration from the preparation walls as excessive leverage may result in cusp/wall fracture. Replacement restorations are subject to the same principles of preparation design and associated operative techniques in their placement as are deployed for primary restorations.

In all cases in which a restoration is to be repaired or replaced, the likely cause of failure should be identified, the preparation modified and, if appropriate, the local environment modified (e.g. by removal of non-working interferences on the tooth/restoration in question) in order to ensure maximum life of the new restoration. In all cases, the preparation should be reassessed to consider its potential for clinical effectiveness, in some cases an extended, indirect or full-coverage restoration may be indicated. Blind repetition of the initial operative approach is likely to be followed by ignominious repetition of failure.

REFERENCES

1. Axelsson P. and Lindhe J. Effect of controlled oral hygiene procedures on caries and periodontal disease in adults. Results after 6 years. *J Clin Periodontol*, 1981; **8**: 239–48.
2. Qvist J., Qvist V. and Mjor I.A. Placement and longevity of amalgam restorations in Denmark. *Acta Odontol Scand*, 1990; **48**: 297–303.
3. Qvist V., Qvist J. and Mjor I.A. Placement and longevity of tooth-colored restorations in Denmark. *Acta Odontol Scand*, 1990; **48**: 305–11.
4. Mjor I.A., Burke F.J. and Wilson N.H.F. The relative cost of different restorations in the UK. *Br Dent J*, 1997; **182**: 286–9.
5. NHS Centre for Reviews and Dissemination. *Undertaking Systematic Reviews of Research on Effectiveness: CRD's Guidance for Carrying Out or Commissioning Reviews*, 2nd edn. NHS Centre for Reviews and Dissemination, University of York, 2001.
6. Ryge G. and Snyder M. Evaluating the clinical quality of restorations. *J Am Dent Assoc*, 1973; **87**: 369–77.
7. Akerboom H.B., Advokaat J.G., Van Amerongen W.E. and Borgmeijer P.J. Long-term evaluation and rerestoration of amalgam restorations. *Community Dent Oral Epidemiol*, 1993; **21**: 45–8.
8. Gruythuysen R.J., Kreulen C.M., Tobi H., van Amerongen E. and Akerboom H.B. 15-year evaluation of Class II amalgam restorations. *Community Dent Oral Epidemiol*, 1996; **24**: 207–10.
9. Djemal S., Setchell D., King P. and Wickens J. Long-term survival characteristics of 832 resin-retained bridges and splints provided in a post-graduate teaching hospital between 1978 and 1993. *J Oral Rehabil*, 1999; **26**: 302–20.
10. Faculty of General Dental Practitioners [FGDP]. Radiographs in dental caries diagnosis. In: *Selection Criteria for Dental Radiography*, 2nd edn. London, FGDP(UK), 2004, pp. 41–52.
11. Valderhaug J., Jokstad A., Ambjornsen E. and Norheim P.W. Assessment of the periapical and clinical status of crowned teeth over 25 years. *J Dent*, 1997; **25**: 97–105.
12. Hunter A.R., Treasure E.T. and Hunter A.J. Increases in cavity volume associated with the removal of class 2 amalgam and composite restorations. *Oper Dent*, 1995; **20**: 2–6.

13. Abou-Rass M. The stressed pulp condition: an endodontic-restorative diagnostic concept. *J Prosthet Dent*, 1982; **48**: 264–7.

14. Paterson F.M., Paterson R.C., Watts A. and Blinkhorn A.S. Initial stages in the development of valid criteria for the replacement of amalgam restorations. *J Dent*, 1995; **23**: 137–43.

15. Mjor I.A. Repair versus replacement of failed restorations. *Int Dent J*, 1993; **43**: 466–72.

16. Mjor I.A. and Gordan V.V. Failure, repair, refurbishing and longevity of restorations. *Oper Dent*, 2002; **27**: 528–34.

17. Cipriano T.M. and Santos J.F. Clinical behaviour of repaired amalgam restorations: a two-year study. *J Prosthet Dent*, 1995; **73**: 8–11.

Evidence based practice

INTRODUCTION – WHAT IS EVIDENCE BASED PRACTICE?

The practice of dentistry is becoming more complex and challenging. Developments in dental materials and techniques, changing socio-demographic patterns, increasingly knowledgeable health care consumers, and the information 'explosion' all place greater demands on clinical decision making. As health care practitioners, it is important to offer the best possible care for patients. However, few decisions made in the health services are made as a result of good evidence. Evidence based practice (EBP) aims to encourage the practitioner to look for, and make sense of, the available research evidence in order to apply it to everyday clinical problems. This presents a challenge to the practitioner as within dentistry alone there are around 500 journals publishing over 43 000 research articles a year. Given that a large proportion of these papers are of limited relevance to everyday practice and often of poor quality, how do you know which of these articles you should read to inform your practice and which you can disregard? You need to be able to identify articles that are both of a high quality and relevant to your clinical practice.

EBP has been defined as 'the conscientious, explicit and judicious use of current best evidence in making decisions about the care of individual patients'[1]. It aims to inform, not replace clinical judgement and experience, by integrating the best evidence with clinical expertise and patient preferences. EBP can be broken down into five key stages, as illustrated in Fig. 8.1. The key stages require the development of skills that encourage the process of life-long learning, allowing the practitioner to identify and react appropriately to emerging information. This chapter will explore, in brief, some of the skills involved in the EBP process.

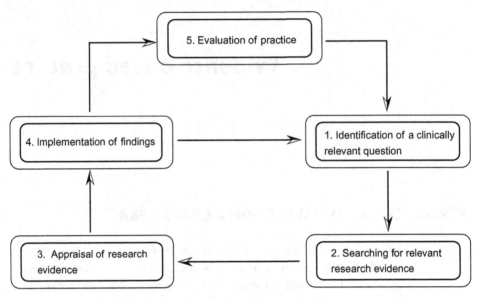

Fig. 8.1 The key stages involved in evidence based practice.

IDENTIFYING AND DEFINING RELEVANT QUESTIONS

Everyday clinical practice can present a vast array of dilemmas regarding the prevention, diagnosis, prognosis or treatment of oral diseases and disorders. EBP encourages the recognition of uncertainty when making clinical decisions. The first step in the EBP process requires the area of clinical uncertainty to be translated into a focused, clinically relevant question.

For example, an adult patient presents with a cavity in a posterior tooth. You explain the different restoration options available to them. They stress that the appearance of the restoration is important to them and that they have heard that ceramic inlays can produce a good colour match with the surrounding tooth. However, they have concerns over the longevity of such restorations in comparison to amalgam and want to know exactly how long they might expect a ceramic inlay to last. You decide to examine the research literature to try and find an answer to their question.

Before looking for relevant information to answer your question, it is a good idea to define your question so that you know exactly what you're looking for. One way to do this is to break it down into sections. Clinical research questions can usually be broken down into the following (PICO) components:

- Population – who are the participants within the study?
- Intervention/Exposure – what are the interventions, risk factors or exposures of interest?
- Comparison – what control comparisons do you want to make?
- Outcomes – what outcome measures are of interest to you and your patient?

Using the previous example, the question you want to answer is 'how effective are ceramic inlays?' Applying the PICO format allows us to define the question further. The patient group **(P)** of interest can be defined as *adults requiring a restoration to any posterior tooth*. The restoration/intervention **(I)** of interest to the patient is *ceramic inlays*. The patient wants to know how long ceramic inlays are likely to last in comparison **(C)** to *amalgam*. The outcomes **(O)** of importance to both you and your patient include the *longevity* of the restoration and *aesthetics*.

Structuring the question in this way can help clarify the type of question you are asking and how to identify the relevant information to answer your question.

IDENTIFYING EVIDENCE

There are a number of sources of information a health professional can turn to in order to find the answer to a question. For example, they may draw upon their own clinical judgement or past experience, they may turn to colleagues for advice, read relevant textbooks or journal articles, search electronic bibliographic databases (e.g. MEDLINE or EMBASE) or secondary sources of information (e.g. *The Cochrane Library, The Journal of Evidence Based Dental Practice, Evidence-based Dentistry*). All of the available sources of information have advantages and disadvantages (Table 8.1).

The ability to carry out quick and reliable searches to identify relevant research evidence is one of the key skills required when practising evidence based dentistry. Before starting to search for research evidence, it is necessary to consider what type of evidence would be most appropriate to answer your research question. Different clinical research questions require evaluation through different study designs. The ceramic inlay example deals with the effectiveness of a treatment option and would be best answered by a randomised controlled trial (RCT) or, ideally, a systematic review of RCTs. However, it must be noted that although RCTs and systematic

Table 8.1 Advantages and disadvantages of different sources of information.

Source	Advantage	Disadvantage
Colleague	Quick response	May be biased May be out of date
Text book	Easy to access	Quickly out of date
Journal article	Full text of recent research	Difficult to access/identify relevant information
Bibliographic databases (e.g. MEDLINE)	Available online Access to large amounts of information Sometimes links to full text online	Can be difficult to search Databases are not comprehensive in their coverage of published journals
Secondary sources (e.g. Systematic Reviews on *The Cochrane Library*)	Provide summaries of relevant research evidence Aim to be unbiased and up to date	Can be difficult to search Do not cover all topics

reviews of RCTs may well be the 'gold standard' upon which to base decisions on the effectiveness of interventions, they are not necessarily appropriate, or ethical, to answer all questions. For example, you may be interested in the prognosis of endodontic treatment in patients with diabetes mellitus. An RCT would obviously not be helpful in answering this question. For questions regarding prognosis such as this, cohort studies would be more appropriate. Table 8.2 illustrates the types of studies designs most suitable for different types of research questions arising in endodontics. The most appropriate source of information will depend upon the type of study design being sought.

For questions regarding the effectiveness of healthcare interventions, the best place to start looking for information is *The Cochrane Library*: http://www.cochrane.org/reviews/clibintro.htm

The Cochrane Library is recognised as the best single source of systematic reviews and controlled clinical trials, covering all aspects of healthcare. It is available through many university libraries and postgraduate centres. It is also freely available to all residents in many countries including the British Isles (a full list of countries with free access is available at http://www.update-software.com/cochrane/provisions.htm).

For questions not focusing on the effectiveness of interventions, other study designs will need to be sought, for which MEDLINE can

Table 8.2 Study designs and the types of questions they address.

Definition of study design	Used for
Experimental studies	
Randomised controlled trial: parallel group design – a group of participants (or other unit of analysis, e.g. teeth) is randomised into different treatment groups. These groups are followed up for the outcomes of interest	Evaluating the effectiveness of an intervention *Randomised controlled trial comparing the longevity and aesthetics of two restorative materials*
Randomised controlled trial: split-mouth design – each patient is his/her own control. A pair of similar teeth, or groups of teeth (quadrants) may be selected and randomly allocated to different treatment groups	*Controlled trial comparing the longevity of simply repairing or replacing restorations*
Non-randomised controlled trial – allocation of participants under the control of the investigator, but the method falls short of genuine randomisation	
Observational studies	
Cohort – a longitudinal study, identifying groups of participants according to their exposure/intervention status. Groups are followed forward in time to measure the development of different outcomes	Measuring the incidence of a disease; looking at the causes of disease; determining prognosis *Cohort study looking at the progress of carious lesions over time and relating this to external factors such as smoking or diet*
Case–control – involves identifying two groups; those who have the outcome of interest (cases) and those who have not (controls). The investigator then looks back in time to see who had the exposure/intervention of interest	Looking at the causes of disease; identification of risk factors; suitable for examining rare diseases *Case–control study comparing patients with endodontic infection (cases) with patients without (controls), looking at associated risk factors*
Cross-sectional survey – the observation of a defined population at a single point in time or time interval. The status of an individual with respect to the presence or absence of both exposure/intervention and outcome are determined at the same time	Measuring the prevalence of a disease; examining the association *Cross-sectional survey of caries in young adults in the North West of England*

be a valuable source. MEDLINE is the US National Library of Medicine's (NLM) premier bibliographic database. It can be accessed free of charge via http://www.ncbi.nlm.gov/PubMed but is also available through other database providers such as Ovid and SilverPlatter.

Searching electronic databases is a complex process, too detailed to cover in this chapter, particularly as databases and service providers all vary in terms of their specific searching 'rules'[2]. However, there are certain elements that should be considered when developing a search strategy for an electronic database which we will cover briefly.

Controlled vocabulary and free text-terms

Many people when searching electronic databases tend to rely on free-text searching; simply typing a phrase, such as 'ceramic inlays', into the search box. The problem that arises when relying on free-text searching is that it depends on finding the exact match of text within the title, abstract (if present) or indexing field of the record. If the author of a study has described the restoration in any way other than 'ceramic inlays', for example 'porcelain inlays', the record will not be retrieved. To help overcome this, many databases use an indexing system for coding records entered onto the database. For example, MEDLINE and *The Cochrane Library* both use MeSH (Medical Subject Headings). All references added onto the database are assigned appropriate MeSH by indexers at the NLM. An example of some dental MeSH terms (section of MeSH Tree) are shown below. The broadest term 'Dentistry, operative' at the top and more specific headings indented below:

- Dentistry, operative
- Crown lengthening
- Dental cavity lining
- Dental restoration failure
- Dental restoration, permanent
  - — Crowns
    - ○ Post and core technique
  - — Inlays
  - — Marginal adaptation (dentistry)
- Dental restoration, temporary
  - — Crowns
    - ○ Post and core technique

It is recommended that a combination of appropriate MeSH and free-text terms be used when searching electronic databases to improve the identification of all relevant research articles.

Search operators and truncation symbols

Most databases allow the combining of search terms using the Boolean operators AND, OR and NOT. The operator AND is used when the research article must contain both search terms, for example 'ceramic' AND 'inlay' (this will reduce the number of articles retrieved). The operator OR is used when either search term is acceptable, for example 'porcelain' OR 'ceramic' (this will broaden the number of articles retrieved). By using NOT between search terms will require the article to contain the first search term but not the second, for example 'restoration' NOT 'crown'. In addition, some databases use proximity operators such as NEAR, NEXT or ADJACENT, which can also be helpful in focusing a search.

Truncation symbols can be used to broaden a search by allowing any ending to a given free-text word. For example, the truncation symbol in *The Cochrane Library* and PubMed is an asterisk. If placed at the end of 'restorat*' this will allow the retrieval of records containing the words restorative, restoration, restorations, restorating, etc. . . . Truncation symbols vary according to databases. When choosing to search a particular database, ensure you are familiar with both the search operators and the truncation symbols available.

If we return to the ceramic inlays example, and acknowledge that the most appropriate database to search initially would be *The Cochrane Library*, we can explore how search results can vary depending upon the approach we take. Table 8.3 shows the results obtained when different free-text terms, MeSH terms, search operators and truncation symbols are used.

The results obtained through searching *The Cochrane Library* (Table 8.3) identified one relevant systematic review, entitled 'Ceramic inlays for restoring posterior teeth'[3]. As systematic reviews provide a comprehensive, objective overview of research in a given area, this would be the obvious article to read first. If such a systematic review did not exist, individual studies of an appropriate study design (in this case RCTs) would have to be examined.

APPRAISAL OF RESEARCH LITERATURE

Let's assume your searching of the literature has identified several relevant primary studies. All the studies use an appropriate study design for answering your research question. Consideration still needs to be given to the fact that within any particular design there is huge variability between studies with regard to how well they are conducted. An important issue to consider at this stage is the study's validity, in particular internal validity.

Table 8.3 Example of results obtained when different free-text terms, MeSH terms, search operators and truncation symbols are used when searching an electronic database (*The Cochrane Library*, Issue 4, 2003).

Term	Number of systematic reviews	Number of controlled clinical trials
Ceramic inlays	1	25
Ceramic inlay	1	7
Ceramic inlay*	1	29
Porcelain inlays	0	4
Porcelain inlay	1	0
Porcelain inlay*	1	4
Ceramic* AND inlay*	1	46
CERAMIC (MeSH)	2	95
INLAYS (MeSH)	1	47
Combining free-text terms and MeSH can help increase the sensitivity and specificity of your search		
(CERAMIC (MeSH) OR ceramic* or porcelain) AND (INLAYS (MeSH) OR inlay*)	1	48

Internal validity refers to the degree to which the results of a study are likely to approximate to the 'truth' for the circumstances being studied[4]. Has the study been conducted in such a way that systematic error (bias) has been minimised? *External* validity refers to the degree to which the effects observed in the study are applicable to the outside world; how generalisable are the results to other circumstances[5]? If internal validity does not exist, there is little point in considering a study's external validity. There are numerous ways in which bias can affect the internal validity of a study. Some of the main biases[6] are described in Table 8.4.

There is a plethora of critical appraisal checklists and resources available. Some guidance on the types of questions to ask[7,8] when reading research articles is presented below:

- What is the research question?
- Is the study design appropriate?
- How well was the study conducted? Consider issues of:
  - Internal validity
  - Sample size
  - Validity of outcome measures
  - Duration of follow-up

Table 8.4 Potential biases affecting the internal validity of a study.

Bias	Definition	Method of overcoming bias
Selection bias	Systematic differences between comparison groups in prognosis or responsiveness to treatment	Randomisation
Performance bias	Systematic differences in care provided to participants in a study, apart from the intervention being evaluated	Blinding of participants and investigators to treatment allocation
Measurement bias	Systematic differences in how outcomes are ascertained from the groups under comparison	Blind outcome assessment
Attrition bias	Systematic differences between comparison groups in withdrawals or exclusions of participants from the results of a study	Intention to treat analysis

- What are the results?
  - — Do the numbers add up?
  - — Are all participants accounted for?
  - — Was the statistical significance assessed?
  - — Were the statistical techniques appropriate?
- What are the implications for practice?

It is acknowledged that this chapter does not cover the critical appraisal of all types of research articles published in the dental literature. For further guidance on how to appraise systematic reviews, clinical guidelines, qualitative research, economic evaluations in addition to the study designs already discussed, the following key resources are recommended:

- Critical Appraisal Skills Programme (*CASP*)
  http://www.phru.nhs.uk/~casp/casp.htm and the *CASP International Network* (a collaboration of individuals and organisations across the world who are interested in helping people develop skills in making sense of scientific evidence – available in Chinese)
  http://www.caspinternational.org.uk/

- The *How to read a paper series* by Trisha Greenhalgh, available online via the *British Medical Journal* website (http://www.bmj.com). The series is also available as a book:
  Greenhalgh T. *How to Read a Paper. The Basics of Evidence Based Medicine*. London, BMJ Publishing Group, 1997.

- The *Users' guide to the medical literature* initially published in the *Journal of the American Medical Association* and available online at http://www.cche.net/usersguides/main.asp. This series has also been updated and published as a book:
  Guyatt G, Rennie D. *Users' Guide to the Medical Literature. A Manual for Evidence-based Clinical Practice*. Chicago, American Medical Association, 2002.

- Crombie I. *The Pocket Guide to Critical Appraisal: A Handbook for Health Care Professionals*. London, BMJ Publishing Group, 1996.

- The Appraisal of Guidelines Research and Evaluation (*AGREE*) instrument provides a framework for evaluating the quality of clinical practice guidelines http://www.agreecollaboration.org/

Often a first attempt at critical appraisal can feel slow and cumbersome, but with practice it becomes rapid and almost automatic. By developing skills associated with critical appraisal healthcare workers will become more adept at managing the ever increasing information overload. It is imperative that any healthcare worker wishing to practise in an evidence based manner develops the ability to quickly identify and interpret high quality, valid and clinically relevant research articles to inform their practice.

IMPLEMENTATION OF RESEARCH EVIDENCE AND EVALUATION OF ITS APPLICATION

Not all valid research articles will be relevant to your clinical practice. Even if a study focuses on a particular intervention or outcome of interest, consideration needs to be given to the external validity of the piece of research. Are the participants included in the research article similar enough to the patients you deal with, or are they so different that the results don't apply? Even if you feel the study is relevant to your clinical practice, implementing the findings is not always easy. There are many barriers that may prevent the integration of research findings into your everyday practice. Time, financial resources and the organisation of the practice in which you work may all prevent the adoption of research evidence[9]. Similarly, opinion leaders within the practice, current beliefs and attitudes regarding treatment options and, increasingly, patients' perceptions about what they consider to be appropriate care all can play their part in preventing best evidence from changing clinical practice.

A variety of implementation strategies have been used to try and improve the uptake of research findings, including educational outreach visits, manual or computerised reminders, interactive educational sessions and audit and feedback. The effectiveness of an implementation strategy appears to be dependent upon individual circumstances, with multifaceted interventions targeting barriers to change being more likely to be effective than a single intervention[5]. There appears to be no single implementation model that can be applied across all settings. Before attempting to change clinical practice, local barriers need to be identified and strategies to overcome them explored.

CONCLUSION

In order for healthcare practitioners to offer the best possible care for their patients they need to practise in an evidence based manner. This involves the development of skills that will enable the practitioner to find and assess emerging information relevant to his particular clinical practice. These skills include forming appropriate questions, searching the literature, appraisal of research papers and the implementation of the findings into everyday practice. This is an ongoing process which will ensure that patients receive the most up-to-date effective care.

REFERENCES

1. Sackett D., Strau S., Richardson W., Rosenberg W. and Haynes R. *Evidence-based Medicine*, 2nd edn. Toronto, Churchill Livingstone, 2000.
2. Bickley S. and Harrison J. How to . . . find the evidence. *J Orthod*, 2003; **30**: 72–78.
3. Hayashi M. and Yeung C. Ceramic inlays for restoring posterior teeth. In: *The Cochrane Library*, Issue 3, 2004.
4. Juni P., Altman D. and Egger M. Assessing the quality of randomised controlled trials. In: Egger, M., Davey Smith, G. and Altman, D. (eds) *Systematic Reviews in Health Care. Meta-analysis in Context*. London, BMJ Publishing Group, 2001, pp. 87–108.
5. NHS Centre for Reviews and Dissemination. *Undertaking Systematic Reviews of Research on Effectiveness: CRD's Guidance for Carrying out or Commissioning Reviews*, 2nd edn. NHS Centre for Reviews and Dissemination, University of York, 2001.

6. Clarke M. and Oxman A. *Cochrane Reviewers' Handbook 4.2.1* [updated March 2004]. In: *The Cochrane Library*, Issue 4, 2004, pp. 49–60.

7. Crombie I. *The Pocket Guide to Critical Appraisal: A Handbook for Health Care Professionals*. London, BMJ Publishing Group, 1996.

8. Greenhalgh T. How to read a paper: getting your bearings (deciding what a paper is about). *BMJ*, 1997; **315**: 243–6.

9. Bero L., Grilli R., Grimshaw J., Harvey, E., Oxman, AD and Thomson MA. Closing the gap between research and practice: an overview of systematic reviews of interventions to promote the implementation of research findings. The Cochrane Effective Practice and Organization of Care Review Group. *BMJ*, 1998; **317**: 465–8.

Index

Page numbers in *italics* refer to figures and those in **bold** to tables.

abscesses 88
absorbent plaques 23
absorbent systems 23
abutment teeth
  elective endodontics 91
  root filled 92
access cavities, endodontic 56–62
  design *57*, 58–9
  objectives 56–8
  preparation form 58
  removal of infected dentine 58–9
  technique 59–62
acrylic resins, temporary crowns 137–8
adhesives
  amalgam restorations 44–5
  indirect restorations 146–7
adrenaline 24, 142
aesthetics
  adhesive restorations 146–7
  restoration materials 131–3
air abrasion, caries removal 36
air-jets 23
airway protection 6–7, 52
alloys
  endodontic instruments 63–4
  intraradicular posts 99
amalgam dowel core (Nayyar core) 48, 95, 115
amalgam inserts (amalgapins) *45*, 46
amalgam marginal angle (AMA) 31
amalgam restorations
  alternative materials 110
  bonding systems 44–5
  core 113, 114–15
  pulp protection 38–9, 40, **41**
  root-filled teeth *94*, 95
  supplementary retention 46, 47–8

amelodentinal junction, caries removal 29–30
analgesia, selective 54
ankylosis, dentoalveolar 86
anterior determinants 10
anterior guidance 10
anticipation 6
antisialogogues 24
apex locators, electronic 67
apical constriction 70
apical disease *see* periapical disease
apical foramen 70
apical preparation 70–2
apical seat (apical box) 71
apical taper 71
appraisal, research literature 167–70
Appraisal of Guidelines Research and
    Evaluation (AGREE) instrument 170
articulating paper 8
aspirators 22
astringent solutions 24
attrition bias **169**
avulsion, tooth 83

bacteria
  cariogenesis 15, 18
  internal root resorption and 85
  microleakage and 37
  pulpal ingress 51
balanced force technique 72
balancing side 9
bases, cavity 37, 39–40, **41**
bevelled shoulder margin *123*, 125
biases 168, **169**
bis-acrylate temporary crowns 138
bitewing radiographs, caries diagnosis
    16–17
Black, G.V. 27
  classification of carious lesions **28**
  placement of margins 31

bonding systems 92
  direct restorations 44–5
  indirect restorations 146–7
Boolean operators 166–7
broken down teeth 110–11
bruxism 130
buccal 13, *14*

calcium hydroxide
  cavity liners 39, 40, **41**, *41*, 43
  inter-appointment, in endodontics 73
  pulp capping 42
  in root resorption 85, 86
  stepwise caries removal 42
canine guidance 10, 130
carbon fibre-reinforced posts 99
Caridex 33–4
caries, dental 14–19
  aetiology 14–15
  cavity preparation and design *see* cavity
    preparation and design
  classification **28**
  diagnosis and assessment 15–17
  preservative management 27
  prevention 18–19
  risk assessment 17–18
  removal techniques 29–30, 33–6
  restoration failure and 153
  restoration margins 150, 157
  stepwise removal 42
Carisolv 34–5
case–control studies **165**
CASP International Network 169
cast posts 99
cavities
  access *see* access cavities, endodontic
  large 109
cavity bases 37, 39–40, **41**
cavity liners 37, 39, 40, **41**
cavity preparation and design 27–36
  alternative preparation methods 33–6
  development of final form 30–2
  gaining access 29
  integrity of the restoration 32
  margin placement 31, *32*, 33
  principles 27–9
  pulp protection 36–43
  removal of caries 29–30
  retentive/resistance features 31–2, 45–6

cavity sealers 37, 38–9, 40, **41**
cavity varnishes 38–9, 40
cavo-surface angle (CSA) 31, *33*
cements
  cavity bases 39, 40
  cavity liners 39
  temporary 138–9
centric
  long/wide 129
  point 129
centric occlusion (CO; intercuspal position)
    8–9
centric relation (CR) 9
ceramic posts 100
ceramic restorations 110
  construction methods 144–5
  factors affecting choice 129–30, 131–2
  margin design 124
  tooth reduction 119
chair
  nurse's 1
  operator's 1
chamfer margin *123*, 125
charting, dental 11–13, *14*
chemomechanical caries removal
    33–5
children, tooth injuries 81, 84
clamps, rubber dam 21–2
clenching habit 130
Cochrane Library 164, 166, 167, **168**
cohort studies 164, **165**
cold sensitivity testing 53
computer-aided design and machining
    (CAD/CAM) techniques 144–5
condylar guidance 10
copal varnish 38
core restorations 111–15
  anterior root-filled teeth 93
  choice of material 114–15
  elective endodontics 91
  materials 113–14
  posterior root-filled teeth 94–100
  space-filling 112
  split 95
  structural *112*, 113
  types 111, *112*
  see also amalgam dowel core; post-core
    restorations
coronal seal, in endodontics 79

costs, economic *see* economic costs
cotton burns 23
cotton wool
    pellets 23
    rolls 23
critical appraisal, research literature
    167–70
Critical Appraisal Skills Programme
    (CASP) 169
cross-sectional surveys **165**
crown (clinical)
    increasing height 147
    surgical lengthening 121, 147
crown-down approach, root canal
    preparation 69
crowns (prosthetic)
    full-coverage 113, 119
    partial-coverage 119
    temporary 136–8
    tooth reduction 119
cuspal protection
    indirect restorations 109, 116
    root-filled teeth 94
cusp fracture
    prevention 109–10, 116
    root-filled teeth 93–4, 109–10

Dahl principle 149
databases, searching electronic 165–7
deciduous dentition *see* primary dentition
delegation 6
dentine
    caries removal 29, 42–3
    desensitisers 39, 40, **41**
    fractures into 83
    infected, access cavities 58–9
    pulp protection 40
dentine bonding agents
    amalgam restorations 38–9, 40
    indications for use 40, **41**
dentine pins 46–8
desensitisers, dentine 39, 40, **41**
determinants of mandibular movements
    10
devitalisation, elective 90–2
    decision making 92
    rationale 90–1
    risks and complications 91–2
diet, caries and 18

direct restorations 27–50
    alternative preparation methods 33–6
    principles 27–32
    pulp protection 36–43
    root-filled teeth 93, *94*, 95
    supplementary retention 43–8
    see also cavity preparation and design
disclusion
    delayed 129
    immediate 129
distal 13, *14*
dressings, temporary 40
dyes, caries diagnosis 16

economic costs
    failed restorations 155
    indirect restorations 150
EDTA 73
elbow 70, *71*
elective endodontics *see* devitalisation,
    elective
electrical conduction methods, caries
    diagnosis 17
electronic apex locators 67
electronic pulp testers 53
electrosurgery 142–3
enamel, chipped 82
endodontic disease *see* pulp disease
endodontic instruments 62–7
    alloys 63–4
    electronic apex locators 67
    hand 64–6
    ISO standardisation 62–3
    rotary 66–7
endodontics 51–80, 81–105
    access cavities 56–62
    cleaning and shaping 68–73
    diagnosis and assessment 52–4
    elective 90–2
    imaging 54–6
    inter-appointment medicaments
        73–5
    obturation 75–9
    perio-endo lesions 86–90
    tooth restoration after 93–100
    in trauma 81–6
ergonomics 1–8
    four-handed dentistry 6–8
    illumination 5–6

ergonomics (cont.)
  operator and nurse positions 2, 3
  operator's chair 1
  patient position 3–5
eugenol based materials
  cavity liners 39
  temporary cements 139
evidence
  identifying 163–7, **168**
  implementing/evaluating application
    170–1
  types 163–4, **165**
evidence based practice (EBP) 161–72
  appraisal of research literature 167–70
  defined 161
  finding the evidence 163–7, **168**
  implementing findings/evaluation
    170–1
  key stages *162*
  posing relevant questions 162–3
examination
  caries 15–16
  charting 11–13, *14*
  dentition 8–13
  occlusion 8–11
excursion/excursive movements 9,
    129–30
experimental studies **165**
extra-coronal restorations 107–8
  tooth reduction 119
  vs intra-coronal 133
eyewear, protective 7

failure, restoration 154–6
  costs to tooth 155–6
  economics 155
  prevention 153–4
  recognition 154–5
feather edge margin 123
Federation Dentaire Internationale (FDI)
  tooth notation system 12–13
ferric sulphate 142
ferrule 122
fibre-optic transillumination, caries
  diagnosis 16
fibre-reinforced posts 99–100
files, endodontic hand 64–6
finishing lines *see* margins
FlexoFiles 66

fluorescence, laser, caries detection 17
fluoride 18–19, 153
four-handed dentistry 6–8
  methods 7–8
  principles 6–7
fractures
  cavity design aspects 30–1
  cusp *see* cusp fracture
  into dentine 83
  exposing pulp 83
  involving crown and root 83
  prevention 30, 109–10, 116
  root *see* root fractures
full-coverage indirect restorations 119

Gates Glidden drills 66
gingivae
  chemical control of exudate/
    haemorrhage 141–2
  electrosurgery 142–3
  management, impression taking
    139–43
  physical retraction 140–1
  rotary curettage 143
gingival sulcus, biological width 147
glass-ionomer cements (GIC)
  cavity bases 40
  cavity liners 39, **41**
  core restorations 114
  resin-modified *see* resin-modified glass-
    ionomer cements
gold cores 113
gold posts 99
gold restorations
  adhesive bonding 146
  factors affecting choice 129–30, 131,
    132
  structural durability 125
  tooth reduction 119
granulomas, periapical/lateral periodontal
  88
greater taper (GT) hand files 66
grinding, tooth 130
grooves
  direct restorations 45, 46
  indirect restorations 121, 145
group function 10, 130
GT (greater taper) hand files 66
guidance 10, 130

gutta-percha 76–7
  sealers 76
  softened filling techniques 78–9
  solid core filling techniques 77–8
gypsum 144

habits, parafunctional 130
hand endodontic instruments 64–6
heat sensitivity testing 53
Hedström files 64–5
home position 4, 5
How to Read a Paper (Greenhalgh) 169
hypnosis 24

illumination 5–6
imaging *see* radiographs
impressions 139–43
  gingival management 139–43
  restoration construction from 143–4
  three-dimensional optical 144
incisal 13
incisal guidance 10
indirect restorations 107–28, 129–52
  categories 107–8
  choice of material 129–33
    aesthetics and patient wishes 131–3
    functional demands 129–30
    space considerations 131
  construction methods 143–5
    computer-aided 144–5
    direct pattern 144
    indirect pattern 143–4
  creation of interocclusal space 147–9
  elective endodontics 90
  full-coverage 119
  impression taking 139–43
  indications 108–11
  intra *vs* extra-coronal 133
  limitations 150
  marginal integrity 122–5
  occlusal stability 126
  partial-coverage 119, 133–4
  preservation of tooth structure 116–19
  principles of preparation 115–26
  retention and resistance 120–1
    limited 145–7
  root-filled teeth 93, 94–5, 109–10, 115
    see also posts, intraradicular

structural durability 125–6
  temporisation 134–9
  see also core restorations
information sources 163, **164**
injection technique, obturation 79
injuries *see* trauma
inlays
  ceramic 110
  protection of tooth structure 116
  resin composite 110
  temporary 135–6
instruments
  endodontic 62–7
  transfer 7–8
intercuspal position (ICP) 8–9
interference 10
International Organization for Standardization (ISO), endodontic instrument standards 62–3
interocclusal space
  creation 147–9
  tooth reduction 131
intra-coronal restorations 107
  vs extra-coronal 133
intra-radicular posts *see* posts, intra-radicular
iodine compounds 73
irrigation, root canal 61, 72, 85

K-Flex files 65
K-type files 65

labial 13
lasers
  caries detection 17
  caries removal 36
lateral condensation technique, obturation 77–8
lateral excursion 9
liners, cavity 37, 39, 40, **41**
lingual 13, **14**
local anaesthesia, caries removal 35
longevity, restoration 153
loose tooth 84
luting cements 120

magnification 6
  caries diagnosis 16
  in endodontics 60

maintenance, restored dentition 153–9
margins
  access cavities 61
  bevelled shoulder 123, 125
  caries at 150, 157
  cavo-surface angle (CSA) 31, 33
  chamfer 123, 125
  direct restorations 31, 32
  feather edge 123
  indirect restorations 122–5
  shoulder 123, 124–5
  sub-gingival 122, 147
master cone radiographs 55–6, 78
materials
  core 113–14
  direct restorations 30
  indirect restorations 129–33
  intraradicular posts 99–100
  root filling 76–7
matrix bands 24
maximum interdigitation position (MIP;
  intercuspal position) 8–9
measurement bias 169
MEDLINE 164–5, 166
MeSH terms 166
mesial 13, 14
metallo-ceramic restorations
  factors affecting choice 132–3
  structural durability 125
  tooth reduction 119
metal restorations
  adhesive bonding 146
  construction 144
  factors affecting choice 129–30, 131,
    132
  margin design 124, 125
  tooth reduction 119
methacrylate temporary crowns 137–8
microleakage 37
mineral trioxide aggregate (MTA) 42,
  75
mirrors 2, 3
models, study 8, 126, 144
moisture control 19–24, 51–2

National Library of Medicine (NLM), US
  165
Nayyar core see amalgam dowel core

nickel titanium 63–4
  hand files 66
  rotary instruments 66–7
non-carious tooth tissue loss (NCTTL)
  146
non-randomised controlled trial 165
non-working contact 10
non-working interference (NWI) 10–11
non-working side 9
nurse, dental
  chair 1
  four-handed dentistry 6–8
  position 2

obturation (root filling) 75–9
  coronal seal 79
  materials 76–7
  objectives 75
  rationale 75
  techniques 77–9
occlusal 13, 14
occlusal vertical dimension (OVD),
  increasing 149
occlusion 8
  examination 8–11
  indirect restorations and 126
operator
  chair 1
  four-handed dentistry 6–8
  position 2
  vision 2, 3
opposing dentition, indirect restorations
  130
oral hygiene 19, 153
orbiting side 9
orthodontics, to create interocclusal space
  148–9

pain 35, 52
palatal 13, 14
Palmer tooth notation system 12
parafunctional habits 130
parallelism 121
partial-coverage indirect restorations 119,
  133–4
patients
  choice of restoration material 131–3
  position 3–5

percussion, tooth 53
performance bias **169**
periapical disease
  assessment 52, 53, 54
  combined periodontal/endodontic
    lesions 88
  pathogenesis 51
periapical radiographs 54–6
  failed restorations 155
  follow-up 56
  master cone 55–6, 78
  preliminary 54–5
  working length estimation 55
periodontal disease 139
  diagnosis 53, 88
  subgingival margins and 147
  vs endodontic disease 88–9
periodontal/endodontic lesions, combined
    86–90
  classifications 87–9
  differential diagnosis 89
  treatment planning 89–90
periodontal ligament
  localised injury 86
  pulp connections 86, 87
periodontitis, apical/lateral 73, 88
pH, caries formation and 15
pharmacological agents, moisture control
    24
PICO components, clinical research
    questions 162–3
plaque, dental 15
Pocket Guide to Critical Appraisal (Crombie)
    170
polymethylmethacrylate temporary
    crowns 137–8
porcelain *see* ceramic
position
  nurse 2
  operator 2
  patient 3–5
post-core restorations 115
  elective endodontics 91
  flow charts 101, 102
  indirect *vs* direct 98, 100
  see also posts, intraradicular
post-crown 96
posterior determinants 10

posterior guidance 10
posts, intra-radicular 95, 96–100
  bridge abutment teeth 92
  design 96–100
  diameter 97
  direct 98, 99, 100
  elective endodontics 91–2
  flow charts 101, 102
  indications 96
  indirect 98, 100
  length 96–7
  materials 99–100
  shape 97–8
  surface finish 98
preservative management 27
primary dentition
  tooth notation 12–13
  traumatic injuries 81, 84
protrusion 9
provisional restorations 135
PubMed 165, 167
pulp
  elective extirpation *see* devitalisation,
    elective
  fractures exposing 83
  periodontal connections 86, 87
  stressed 90, 155–6
pulp capping 42–3
  direct 42
  indirect 42–3
pulp chamber
  entry into 59
  roof removal 59–61
pulp disease
  clinical features 52
  pathogenesis 51
  vs periodontal disease 88–9
pulp protection 36–43
  current concepts 37–40
  historical concepts 37
  indications 40–2
pulp vitality testing 52–4
  combined endodontic/periodontal
    lesions 89
  traumatic injuries 82

quadrants 11–12
questions, clinical research 162–3

radiographs
  caries diagnosis 16–17
  endodontic 54–6
  failed restorations 155
  traumatic injuries 82
randomised controlled trials (RCTs) 163–4,
  165
rationalisation 6
reamers 64
recapitulation 72
refractory die 144
reimplantation, avulsed tooth 83
repair, restoration 156–8
replacement, failed restorations 156–8
resin adhesives 44, 146
resin composite
  core restorations 113–14, 115
  indirect restorations 110
    adhesive bonding 146
    construction 144
  pulp capping 42
  pulp protection 38, 39, **41**
  root-filled teeth 93, *94*
  supplementary retention methods 47
  temporary crowns 138
resin-modified glass-ionomer cements
  cavity liners 39, *41*
  core restorations 95, 114
  root-filled teeth 79, 93, *94*
resistance 120
  direct restorations 43–8
  indirect restorations 121, 145–7
resorption, traumatised teeth *see* root
    resorption
restoration materials *see* materials
restorations
  direct *see* direct restorations
  failure 154–6
  indirect *see* indirect restorations
  maintenance 153–4
  replacement and repair 156–8
  survival time 153
retention
  amalgam dowel core 48
  bonding methods 44–5
  dentine pins 46–8
  direct restorations 31–2, 43–8
  indirect restorations 120–1, 145–7
  preparation design features 45–6

retraction cord, gingival 140–1
retruded axis position (RAP) 9
retruded contact position (RCP) 9
retrusion 9
root canals
  anatomy 57
  cleaning and shaping 68–73
    apical preparation 70–2
    balanced force technique 72
    coronal two-thirds shaping *62*, 69
    mid-third shaping 72
    negotiation of coronal two-thirds 69
    objectives 68
    patency filing 72
    smear layer management 73
    stages 68–9
    working length determination 55,
      69–70
  filling *see* obturation
  instruments *see* endodontic instruments
  inter-appointment medicaments 73–5
  orifice opening 61–2
  see also endodontics
root-filled teeth 93–100
  anterior, restoration 93, *94, 102*
  indirect restorations *see under* indirect
    restorations
  posterior, restoration 93–100, *101, 102*
  strength 91–2, 93, 109–10
root fractures
  endodontically-treated teeth 92
  intra-radicular posts and 96, 98, 99–100
  traumatic 83
root perforation, repair 75
root resorption 85–6
  cervical 85
  external inflammatory 86
  internal 85
  replacement 86
rosin varnish 38
rotary endodontic instruments 66–7
rotary gingival curettage 143
rubber dam 19–22
  clamps 21–2
  endodontics 52, 59
  retention methods 20

safety 6–7
saliva 18

saliva ejectors 22
sealers
   cavity 37, 38–9, 40, **41**
   root canal 76
searching electronic databases 165–7, **168**
   controlled vocabulary *vs* free text 166
   operators and truncation symbols 166–7
selection bias **169**
selective analgesia testing 54
shoulder margin *123*, 124–5
silicone index 118
single cone method, obturation 77
slide 9
slip joint principle 123
smear layer, in endodontics 73
socio-economic status, caries and 18
sodium hypochlorite (NaOCl) 61, 85
sonic instruments, cavity preparation 35
space, interocclusal *see* interocclusal space
splinting, traumatised teeth 84
split core 95
sports, contact 81
spreader 71, 78–9
stainless steel, endodontic instruments 63,
   64, 66
standardisation 6
step-down (step-back) technique, root canal
   preparation 68, 69, 71–2
Stephan curve 15
steroid–antibiotic compounds, in
   endodontics 73
stressed pulp syndrome 90, 155–6
study designs 163–5
surgical crown lengthening 121, 147
systematic reviews 163–4, 167

taper, indirect restorations 120–1
team working *see* four-handed dentistry
temporary cementation 138–9
temporary crowns 136–8
   custom-made 137–8
   prefabricated 136–7
temporary dressings 40
temporary inlays 135–6
temporary restorations 134–9
   indications 134
   vs provisional restorations 135
terminal hinge axis 9
thermal pulp tests 53

tooth
   avulsion 83
   broken down/worn 110–11
   dimensions 68
   fractures *see* fractures
   loose 84
   notation systems 11–13
   strength, minimising effect on 30
   surfaces 13, *14*
   trauma *see* trauma
tooth structure
   loss, restoration failure 155
   preservation of integrity 30–1, 116–19
   reduction, for indirect restoration
      117–19
transfer zone 7
transillumination 16, 54
trauma 81–6
   developing teeth 84
   effects 81–2
   gingival, impression taking 141
   history 82
   prevention 81
   root resorption after 85–6
   splinting 84
   treatment options 82–4
truncation search symbols 166–7
tug-back 77

ultrasonically powered instruments, in
   endodontics 60–1
undercuts 45
universal tooth notation system 13
Users' Guide to the Medical Literature
   (Guyatt & Rennie) 170

validity
   external 168
   internal 167–8, **169**
varnishes, cavity 38–9, 40
veneers, tooth reduction 119
vision, operator's 2, *3*
visual examination, caries 15–16
vitality testing *see* pulp vitality testing

warm lateral condensation method,
   obturation 78–9
warm vertical condensation method,
   obturation 79

wear
    adhesively retained restorations 146
    choice of restoration material and
        129–30
    prevention 116
working length determination 55, 69–70
working side 9

worn teeth 110–11
wrought posts 99

zinc oxide eugenol 40
zinc phosphate cements 40
zinc polycarboxylate 40
zip 70, 71